Fundamentals of Diabetes: Questions and Answers

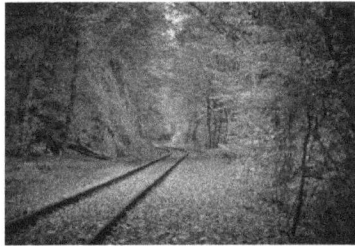

Shunzhong Shawn Bao, M.D.
Endocrinology/Diabetes Specialist

Publisher's Note: The information contained herein is not intended to replace the services of a trained health professional or to be a substitute for individual medical advice. You should consult with your health care professional in regard to any matter relating to your health, and in particular, any matter that may require diagnosis or medical attention.

Uncontrolled high or low blood sugar levels are dangerous, and you need to seek immediate medical care for these conditions. If you are being treated for diabetes, any changes in your existing medications are not advised without first consulting a medical professional. Additionally, any changes in your diet and exercise practices should follow the guidelines of a medical professional who has personally examined you.

Essential Diabetes Questions and Answers:

Shunzhong Shawn Bao, M.D.
Barbara Winter, Editor

Dedication

This book is dedicated to my patients; these are their intelligent questions, for which I am grateful. So many have overcome the seemingly impossible and reversed their diabetes. Their stories have encouraged and inspired me to write this book. This book is for them, my patients.

This book is also dedicated to readers of the first edition. Thank you for your encouragement and support. Your positive feedback urged me to make this book better and to make a larger impact on more patients.

This book is dedicated to my best friend and editor Barbara Winter. With her patience and critiques, she has improved the readability of this book.

I want to thank all the scientists who make the discoveries that I have not mentioned. Without your work, diabetes would still be a desperate disease. Now, because of you, the future for diabetes is so much brighter. I believe that one day we can prevent or cure diabetes. This book is intended to spread your research and your studies.

Finally, this book is dedicated to my wife who deserves deep, enduring gratitude, and also to my two children who are both in medical school. They are "first round editors". They helped me despite their heavy medical school work. They inspire me to learn and strive for excellence in patient care.

Preface

This book is an update to and selection of the most essential questions from my previous book: *Diabetes Questions and Answers: More Than 400 Diabetes Frequently Asked Questions*. The book has had overwhelming positive reviews from patients and readers, so I have made it more concise and more affordable.

Diabetes is a life-long disease, and it is a patient's disease. It is you, the patient, who has to manage your diabetes every day. You do not have off days or vacations. Everyday you encounter new situations. You may ask yourself, what should I do? This book, *Fundamentals of Diabetes: Questions and Answers* makes your job easier.

In this book, I provide an easy to follow road map for you to get your diabetes under control and even reverse the disease. Even if you know when to take or not take your medications, you may still have questions about the side effects and how to reduce them. You may also have questions about how to manage your diabetic neuropathy, sexual dysfunction, and a whole range of health issues related to diabetes. After reading *Fundamentals of Diabetes: Questions and Answers* you will know what your sugar, cholesterol, and blood pressure targets, etc., are. Certainly, you will feel more confident about taking care of yourself.

For most people, a trip to a doctor's office means spending time traveling from out of town and sitting in a crowded waiting room. Imagine that you are a patient who has traveled a few hours to see your doctor, but he or she is only able to spend a few minutes with you.

What if it were possible for you to spend hours with an expert doctor who has worked with diabetic patients for years? What if you could pick his brain to find all the nuggets of wisdom he has learned from treating his diabetic patients? What questions would you ask him?

This book provides you with a treasure trove of information about practical day-to-day solutions for patients living with and managing diabetes. It condenses hundreds of questions and answers into one useful book.

Shunzhong Shawn Bao, MD

Comments from my patients and Amazon.com readers

"The book is so easy to read, and the information is just what I want to know about diabetes."

"The book is just like you are talking to me. Now I have the book, just like I bring you home with me. When I have a question, I can ask at anytime. The answers are so specific and practical."

"...this book is an absolute MUST have for anyone who has diabetes or family/friends with diabetes. It has virtually every question and answer that you could think of for someone with diabetes. I highly recommend this book!!!! "

"...It's not easy, but if you follow Dr Bao's advice, you can lose a lot of weight and get off your medications. It all depends on how bad you want it. Breaks it all down in easy to understand wording. Great book! It is helping me save my life!"

"...I learned so much from reading this book! It was easy to understand and I especially enjoyed all of the information regarding how to cook healthy and how to make the right food choices. My Mom is a type 2 diabetic and she needs help understanding how to manage her diabetes with food and medicines. Super helpful book to achieve this goal! Definitely worth buying and reading!"

"The author uses layman language to answer many of the questions that are frequently asked by diabetic patients. This book is a good resource of information not only for patients with diabetes, but also for people who take care of diabetic patients and who want to prevent diabetes."

"This is a great resource for not only patients with diabetes, but also their families. The book is very easy to follow, and there's so much information that you could not possibly get it all from your doctor."

Contents

Chapter 1: Essentials you need to know after being newly diagnosed with diabetes

Diet and exercise questions

What can I eat?

The first thing people with a new diagnosis of diabetes ask is, "What can I eat?"

My patients know that diet is crucial in controlling diabetes.

I put this list together. Many of my patients like it.

Stay away from:	Recommended:
all fruit juices and soft drinks	water, green tea, black coffee, 1% milk, soy milk, almond milk
pizza, tacos, chips, pretzels, chicken nuggets	salad without dressing, tuna, turkey, chicken
processed meat sausage, hamburgers, hot dogs	real meat chicken breast, turkey breast, fish
red meat	lean cuts fish- salmon, tilapia, mackerel, shrimp
egg yolks	egg whites
potatoes	broccoli, cauliflower, peppers, green beans, kale, cabbage
white bread, pasta, noodles, white rice	whole grains, all beans, shirataki noodles, chia, flaxseeds, quinoa

Stay away from:	Recommended:
watermelon, pineapple, grapes raisins, pawpaws, mangos	all berries-raspberries, cranberries, blackberries, blueberries, strawberries, papayas, apples, cantaloupe (some are too sweet). bananas, kiwi, plums, tangerines, cherries, figs, pomegranates (control portion sizes)
snacks-avoid if possible if sugar is not low candy, ice-cream, honey, chocolate, cookies, pizzas, chicken nuggets	raw or dry roasted nuts-peanuts, almonds, cashews, pistachios, sunflower seeds, pumpkin seeds, Sugar-free Jello, 4-ounce plain or sugar-free yogurt, mushrooms, raw veggies (celery, broccoli), tomatoes, fruit (see above)
candies, ice-cream, cake, cookies	protein bars, nut bars, cheese
pancakes, fried eggs, bacon	oatmeal, egg whites, low carb yogurt
butter	vegetable oil, olive oil
fried food	grilled, baked, broiled, boiled, steamed

The key is three lows: low carbs, low meat, and low calories. Snacking is not recommended. Fruits need to be reduced.

How should I eat?

You should always eat something with fiber at every meal. Eat your food with fiber first. Eat your colorful vegetables before anything else. Eat your food slowly and mindful. Try not to eat snacks, but if your next mealtime is more than five hours away, eat a light snack. Try not to eat snacks just before bed. Drink plenty of water to keep yourself well hydrated.

What can I drink? How much do I need to drink?

I recommend you drink at least 46-64 oz of fluids daily. Water is the best. I do not recommend ice-cold water. It is better warm or room temperature which can soothe your stomach too. Green tea, or black coffee is acceptable. Vitamin water, other flavored waters are okay. Ideally, I prefer products do not have artificial flavor. You can add some fruits to flavor your water.

You should **stay away** from

- fruit juices-even 100%
- soda even diet
- alcohol based drinks like beer
- sweetened tea
- sweetened soy milk or almond milk

You need to reduce milk or milk-based drinks.

What can I do for exercise?

The current recommendation is that you need to have moderate intensity aerobic exercise for 30 minutes a day, 5 days a week. I recommend you have exercise every day.
Here are eight exercise recommendations:

1. Start walking if you can. Get yourself a pedometer, or use an app on your smartphone, Apple Watch or Fitbit, and many others. The point of a step counter is to track your progress, encourage yourself, and keep yourself accountable. Your goal is 10,000 to 15,000 steps a day. Be aware that tracking miles is more accurate than steps. I recommend you walk 3-5 miles a day.

2. If you can stand, do not sit. We all sit too much and sitting is a killer. If possible, you can buy a standing desk so you can stand and work on your computer, or get yourself a treadmill desk (yes, there is a desk with a treadmill). You can walk while working on your computer.

3. Keep moving if you can. Moving is always better than sitting.

4. Choose an activity you like. Think back to your childhood for sports you enjoyed and pick them up again if you can. If this was a team sport, look around and ask your friends and

family if there is a team you can join. You can also look on the internet for interest groups to join.

5. Always start slow and increase activity gradually, especially if you have not been active for a long time. It may take some time for you to build strength.

6. Listen to your body. Stop activity if you have severe shortness of breath, chest pain, or any pain anywhere. You may need to call your doctor to have your heart, lungs or joints evaluated.

7. Ideally, you can join a gym and get a qualified trainer. Most of the time, if you pay money, you will be incentivized to exercise more, because you'll want to get your money's worth.

8. If you like dancing, find an interesting group, so you do not have to be in the gym. If you do not like it, you can learn something new like Taiqi or Yoga.

9. Read my other book on revert prediabetes, diabetes and weight loss.

What exercise should I not do if I go to the gym?

- Do not run on a treadmill.
- Do not lift weight, especially excessive weight.

I have so many people who started very zealous for exercise and hurt their knees, back and so on.

How much weight should I lose?

Any weight loss is helpful. 5-10% can be your initial target. I have a patient who lost half of her body weight and was able to stop all her medications for diabetes, blood pressure and cholesterol.

How fast should I lose weight?

I recommend 1 lb a week. If too fast, you are going to get rebound. Any measures you are using to lose weight, if not sustainable are not going to work. I also recommend you weigh yourself every day. The more attention you pay to your weight, the better you will be.

A1c questions

Diabetes patients are talking about A1c. What is it?

A1c is short for HbA1c, which measures a 2-3 month average of blood sugar. We usually check it every 2-3 months. Sometimes we check it more often if a patient's blood sugar is too high and under active treatment adjustment.

	HbA1C	Average Blood Glucose Level	
	Test Score	Mg/dl (US)	mmol/L
Action Needed	14.0	380	21.1
	13.0	350	19.3
	12.0	315	17.4
	11.0	280	15.6
	10.0	250	13.7
	9.0	215	11.9
OK	8.0	180	10.0
Good	7.0	150	8.2
Excellent	6.0	115	6.3
	5.0	80	4.7
	4.0	50	2.6

.

Blood sugar monitoring questions

How often and when should I check my sugar?

I make these recommendations based on the treatment regimen.

Once a day schedule

No diabetes medications and just diet and exercise. We recommend checking just once a day or 1-2 times a week if you are very stable. You can also somedays check the morning sugar, somedays check the bedtime sugar and somedays check the 2 hours after the meal.

If you are on oral medications, <u>except</u> sulfonylureas (most common are glimepiride, glipizide, glyburide), or glinides (most common are Starlix, Prandin), then you also need to check once a day. You should follow the previous schedule.

Twice a day schedule

If you are on sulfonylurea or glinides, I recommend checking your sugar two times a day.

Fasting and bed time
somedays before the meal and 2 hours after the meal.

Morning and bedtime schedule

If you have basal insulin like Levemir, NPH, Lantus (or Basaglar), Tresiba, or Toujeo, you need to check morning and bedtime. If your A1c is still not reaching your target, then I recommend checking after meals also. You do not have to check every meal but alternating between meals.

If you sugar are stable, it is acceptable that somedays you check the morning sugar, and some days you check the night sugar.

Four times a day schedule

If you are taking multiple shots a day, you need to check sugar at least 4 times a day.

If you have type 1 diabetes, check at least 4 times a day as above. For type 1 diabetes, do additional tests under these circumstances:
- Check whenever you feel your sugar might be high or low.
- Check anytime when you do not feel well.

- Check before you drive.
- Check before and after you exercise to see how you respond to the exercise.
- Also check your urine ketones whenever you do not feel well.

Seven times a day pregnancy schedule

If you are pregnant, you need to check 7 times a day.

Before each meal, 2 hours after the meal and at the bedtime.

Questions about glucometers and continuous glucose monitors (CGM)

I have financial difficulties. What can I do to lower my cost for strips?

You can try Wal-Mart brand (ReliOn). Sometimes, Amazon or other online vendors sell so much cheaper.

Insulin pump and monitoring questions

When should I look into CGM (continuous glucose monitoring)?

Anybody who can afford or whose insurance pays for a CGM is recommended to have one. This is my recommendation.

Which CGM is the best?

In the US, we currently have three CGM systems:
- Medtronic Guardian Connect CGM-FDA approved in March 2018
- Dexcom G6 FDA approved in March 2018
- Freestyle Libre FDA approved at the end of 2017
- Eversense CGM approved in June 2018 for three months use.

I am waiting to try Eversense CGM.

The Medtronic Gaudian Connect CGM is nice because it does not need a receiver. It incorporated with iPhone or iWatch. The data

7

goes to the cloud automatically. You can share your data with other people easily. It is integrated with another app Sugar IQ which can assist patient to dose insulin.

Dexcom G6. It is so much easier compared to Dexcom G5. It is also like Freestyle Libre, no pricking, no calibration. It is so much easier to start and only need 2 hours warm up. It gives you alarms if your sugar is too high or too low. You need an app-Dexcom G6 to collect, view and share the data.

Freestyle Libre is a new device FDA approved in late 2017. The biggest advantage is that you do not need to prick yourself anymore. Lots patients do not check their sugar due to pain or cumbersome. This Freestyle Libre, you can check at any time, and as many times as you want. However, it does not give you alarm if your sugar is too low or too high. Now the warm up time is one hour and the sensor last 14 days. You need an app-Freestyle libreLink to use the iPhone or Android to scan and share. You certainly can use a standalone scanner and upload to LibreView and share with your doctor.

Eversense CGM is the first FDA approved 3-month sensor. A small sensor is implanted, and data are transferred to smart phone such as iPhone or iWatch (for compatible devices please consult the Eversense website) and then store in the cloud and can be shared and analyzed. The advantage is that it lasts for three months and will not fall since it is implanted. The disadvantage is that you need to implant it and you still need to calibrate 2 times a day.

If you are tech savvy and insurance pays, I recommend Dexcom G6. If not, I recommend Freestyle Libre. I do not recommend stand-alone Medtronic sensor for my patients since it is complicated and still needs two times fingerstick calibrations every day. I have not tried Eversense CGM. I think I would recommend to only two groups of patients, patients who are allergic to the adhesions; patients who are sweat so much that the sensor cannot be stick on.

Which strips can the Freestyle Libre reader use to check regular finger stick?

The Precision Neo strips can be used with Freestyle Libre reader.

Can I use the CGM while having MRI/CT/Xray?

No, you should not wear CGM sensor while having MRI/CT/Xray. Eversense sensor needs to be removed also.

Blood sugar, cholesterol and weight targets

What sugar target should I shoot for?

Different patients have different targets.
I have more detailed explanation and target setup in my other book <<All about insulin>>.

Normal Target for young otherwise "healthy" patients:
➢ Fasting and before meals: 70-100 mg/dl
➢ 2 hour after meal: <140 mg/dl
➢ A1c target <5.5%

Very Tight Control Target for young otherwise "healthy" but less motivation and less means:
➢ Fasting and before meals: 70-110 mg/dl
➢ 2 hours after meal <140 mg/dl
➢ A1c of 6.0%

Tight Control Target for most diabetes:
➢ Fasting and before meals: 70-120 mg/dl
➢ 2 hours after meal <140 mg/dl
➢ A1c of 6.5%

Conventional Control Target (American Diabetes Association - ADA target) patients less motivation and less means:
➢ Fasting and before meals: 70-140 mg/dl
➢ 2 hours after meals <180 mg/dl
➢ A1c < 7.0%

Reasonable Control Target for patients with low sugars
➢ Fasting and before meals: 70-160 mg/dl, occasionally reaching 180 mg/dl
➢ 2 hours after meals <200 mg/dl

➤ A1c < 8.0%

No Extreme Target elderly not motivated, dementia, limited life expectancy, or very fragile sugar:

➤ Fasting and before meals: 70-200, very rarely to 300
➤ 2 hours after meals <300 mg/dl
➤ No A1c target

Pregnant Target:

➤ Fasting, premeal, bedtime, and overnight glucose: 60-99 mg/dl
➤ After meal 100-120 mg/dl
➤ A1C ≤6%

Your target can be changed.

What is my cholesterol target level?

Every diabetic: below 100 mg/dl, ideally below 70 mg/dl.

If you have a history of one of the following conditions, your LDL target should be below 70 mg/dl or lower.

- myocardial infarction (heart attack)
- angioplasty
- bypass
- stable and unstable angina
- stroke
- TIA (transient ischemic attack)
- carotid endarterectomy or carotid artery over 50% blockage
- other artery procedures-like iliofemoral stents or bypass

If you have one of the following conditions, 2017 AACE guideline called to get LDL below 50 mg/dl.

- Continue to have unstable angina even LDL<70 mg/dl
- Atherosclerotic disease in combination of diabetes, renal failure stage ¾, or FH (familial hypercholesterolemia)

- History of premature atherosclerotic disease (male < 55 years old, female < 65 years old)

What should my blood pressure target be?

It is very important to control your blood pressure. Controlling your blood pressure can protect your kidneys, heart, eyes, and brain. Your blood pressure needs to be controlled under 140/90, ideally below 130/80. 2017 ACC/AHA (American College of Cardiology/American Heart Association) has defined normal blood pressure as below120/80 based on new data. Therefore, if possible, you should get your blood pressure to normal.

Chapter 2: 10 questions to ask your insurance company about diabetes coverage

Currently, insurance companies do not allow doctors to decide many important decisions about your diabetes treatment. The first thing you need to do after you receive your diabetes diagnosis is to call your insurance company. These are the 10 questions you are going to ask.

Does my insurance policy cover diabetes self-management education?

Does my insurance company sponsor any community programs for healthy lifestyle changes?

What kind of glucometer does it cover?

What diabetes medications are in the formulary?

What cholesterol medications does it cover?

Does my insurance cover ophthalmologist's (eye doctor) visits?

Does my insurance cover podiatrist's (foot doctor) visits?

Does my insurance cover weight loss?

Does my insurance cover continuous glucose monitoring (CGM)?

Does my insurance cover insulin pumps?

Chapter 3: 10 things to discuss with your family about diabetes

Diabetes is not an easy condition to deal with. It is a lifelong disease, and it is not a disease that can be cured by a medication or a procedure. It takes lifelong self-management and lifestyle change. You will need a strong support system.

When should I share my diabetes diagnosis with my family and friends?

You need to tell your family as soon as possible.

What should I let my family know about my diet?

Share this booklet with your family.

What should I let my family know about my drinks?

Do not drink anything with calories and cut down "zero" calorie soda.

What does my family need to know about exercise?

Inspire your family member to have exercise today. If you are not exercising with a family member, you need to let your family know where you are exercising and how long. This is important because hyperglycemia (high blood sugar) and hypoglycemia (low blood sugar) can happen, and it is dangerous when they do.

What does my family need to know about my new routine?

Dealing with diabetes can be a full-time job. Getting your family involved can help you do the job better and safer.

What does my family need to know about diabetes medications?

The name of the medication and the dose
When you should take it
What side effect

How do my family and I know if I have low blood sugar?

Educate your family about low sugar. Most patients have weakness, hunger, blurry vision, tremors, palpitations, irritability and sweating and if severe enough, a patient can pass out. Some patients can have mood changes and others behave weirdly or have slurred speech.

Should I teach my family members how to check my sugar?

This is important. Sugar too high or too low can debilitate you. You need help from time to time. Let them know where you keep all the supplies.

How should my family handle glucagon shots?

Review with your family where it is kept, when to use one and how to use it. This can only be used when you are not able to eat or drink anything to raise your sugar. Give the shot first and then call 911 as soon as possible.

Do I need to tell my family about A1c and what my A1c target is?

You should tell them what your A1c target is and how you are planning to reach your target

Chapter 4: 10 questions to ask before starting a new medication

What is the necessity of starting a new medication?

Does it have a generic version?

How will it help my diabetes?

Does it have interactions with other medications I am taking?

What side effects do I need to watch for?

When should I stop or adjust the dose?

Should I take my medications before a meal, with a meal, or after a meal, or at bedtime?

Can I double my dose if my sugar is too high?

Can I continue my medication if I am going to have a CT scan or cardiac catheterization?

What should I do if I am going to have a procedure like a colonoscopy or surgery?

Chapter 5: The basic knowledge of diabetes

Questions about the different types of diabetes

What is diabetes?

Strictly speaking, diabetes is really not a diagnosis. It is a sign. Diabetes used to mean sugar was present in the urine, but now we understand that sugar is too high in the blood. Many reasons can cause high sugar, therefore, there are many types of diabetes.

What is insulin resistance?

It simply means that insulin is not working as efficiently as it should be. Insulin is the hormone that allows sugar to enter cells and tissues such as fat cells or muscle cells where it is metabolized. Many conditions can cause insulin resistance, such as stress, being overweight, or taking some medications.

What is prediabetes?

Blood sugar is not normal, but it does not reach the diagnosis of diabetes yet. Specifically,
- fasting sugar between 100-125 mg /dl
- oral glucose testing, 2-hour sugar between 140-199
- HbA1c is between 5.7%-6.4%.

People with prediabetes can develop complications also.

What is type 1 diabetes?

Type 1 diabetes is the autoimmune destruction of pancreatic beta cells causing insufficient insulin. Generally speaking, if the patient has type 1 diabetes, insulin is required, otherwise, the patient will die. Not all diabetes treated with insulin is type 1 diabetes. For patients who developed diabetes before they were 19 years old, two-thirds of them are type 1 diabetics. Clinically, you can consider any diabetes which is prone to develop DKA (diabetic ketoacidosis) or has a history of DKA as type 1 diabetes. This is really what matters when we are talking about type 1 or type 2 diabetes.

What is type 2 diabetes?

Type 2 diabetes is the most common type of diabetes. About 90% of diabetes in adults is type 2 diabetes, while 30% of diabetes in children is type 2 diabetes. Blood sugar is high because the body cannot use insulin properly, which is called insulin resistance. At the early stages, the pancreas increases insulin secretion to make up for insulin insensitivity for the high blood sugar, but later the pancreas can fail too, which makes the diabetes worse.

What is type 3 diabetes?

Type 3 diabetes is a title that has been proposed for Alzheimer's disease which results from resistance to insulin in the brain. This has not been a broadly accepted concept yet. People who have insulin resistance, in particular, those with type 2 diabetes, have an estimated 50% to 65% risk of suffering from Alzheimer's disease.

What is type 1.5 diabetes?

In the late 1990's, some researchers coined the term "Type 1.5 diabetes," because it had features of the two major types of diabetes. They have both autoimmune destruction of pancreatic beta islet cells and insulin resistance. These patients are adults who at the beginning were more like type 2 diabetes because they could be treated with diet, exercise, and oral medications. They also have type 1 features with autoimmune destruction of the pancreatic beta cells. They also have autoimmune antibodies like the GAD antibody. Later, most of these patients need insulin. We also call them "latent autoimmune diabetes of adults" (LADA). Due to the destruction of beta cells, most of them need insulin later. Now, most doctors classify them as type 1 diabetes.

What is LADA?

"Latent autoimmune diabetes of adults(LADA) is also referred to as type 1.5 diabetes. These patients have autoimmune antibodies like GAD antibody, which indicates that their immune system is attacking their pancreatic beta islet cells. Later most patients need insulin. In the clinic, LADA is treated the same as type 1 diabetes.

Patients with LADA are more stable because they do not easily develop diabetic ketoacidosis (DKA) and severe hypoglycemia.

What is gestational diabetes?

Pregnant women who have never had diabetes before but who have high blood sugar levels during pregnancy are said to have gestational diabetes. People who have gestational diabetes will have a higher risk for developing diabetes after their pregnancies. Pregnant patients with diabetes before they get pregnant are called Diabetes in Pregnancy. Both of these types of diabetes need to be well managed.

Can adults have type 1 diabetes?

Yes, adults can develop type 1 diabetes too. Most commonly, this is in the form of the type 1.5 diabetes, LADA, which is technically type 1 diabetes.

Are there any other types of diabetes?

Technically speaking, the diagnosis of diabetes is not even a diagnosis. It is just a symptom or sign, which means high sugar in the urine (now blood). Many conditions can cause high sugar in the urine and blood. Therefore, there are many types of diabetes. However, for most people, type 1 diabetes, type 2 diabetes, or gestational diabetes are the diagnoses.

What is steroid induced diabetes?

Since the 1940s, steroids have been increasingly used in treating many autoimmune and non-autoimmune diseases. Steroid-induced diabetes is an abnormal increase in blood sugar associated with the use of glucocorticoids in a patient without a prior history of diabetes mellitus.

What is "brown diabetes"?

There is a hereditary single gene disease called hemochromatosis. It causes increased iron absorption and deposition in organs like the pancreas and liver, which causes organ damage, and thus diabetes. The iron deposited in the skin causes it to look brown.
Early diagnosis of hemochromatosis is very important. Your doctor uses blood cell counts, iron tests, and sometime gene tests to make

the diagnosis. Therapeutic phlebotomy is the treatment for hemochromatosis.

What is MODY?

MODY stands for maturity-onset diabetes of the young is caused by a single gene mutation. 3- 5% of all diabetes cases may be due to MODY.

There are eleven different types of MODY caused by changes in eleven different genes. Not all MODYs are the same. Treatment varies, depending on the type of MODY. The complications are the different.

Why are we care to make the diagnosis of MODY?

1) MODY 2 is very mild and usually do not have severe complications. Diet and exercise are the main recommendation.
2) MODY 1, 3, and 4 can usually be managed with a type of medicine called sulfonylurea therapy. Patients can be missed as type 1 or type 2 diabetes. It will be thrilled to both doctor and patients if insulin can be stopped and just take one pill a day.
3) MODY 5 often needs a variety of treatments because it may cause other medical problems unrelated to the blood sugar level..

Questions about other causes of diabetes

Do night shifts cause diabetes?

Yes.

Do sugary drinks really cause diabetes?

Yes.

Do plastic products cause diabetes?

Yes.

Questions about diagnosing diabetes

What are the symptoms of diabetes?

For type 2 diabetes, the most common symptoms are **no symptoms**. Therefore, blood tests are important if you suspect that you have diabetes.
Some symptoms are:

- excessive thirst
- excessive urination
- weight loss (type 1)
- weight gain (type 2)
- blurry vision
- tingling, pain, or numbness in the hands and feet

Why does my doctor say I have diabetes, but I do not have any symptoms?

The most common symptoms of diabetes are no symptoms. The diagnosis of diabetes is made by blood tests.

How is diabetes diagnosed?

A diabetes diagnosis is made by blood tests, although it is semi-arbitrary. We have four ways to make the diagnosis:

1. Fasting sugar 126 mg/dl or greater twice
2. At any time the sugar 200 mg /dl or greater and you have some sort of diabetes symptoms
3. Oral sugar testing-OGTT, 2-hour sugar is 200 mg/dl or greater
4. HbA1c 6.5% or greater

Questions about doctors and doctor's visits

What are some questions I should ask my doctor about diabetes treatment?

You can ask your doctor any of the questions in this book. For every visit, you need to prepare yourself. You need to know your A, B, C, D, E and Fs.

A stands for A1c.
B stands for blood pressure.
C stands for cholesterol.
D stands for drugs (medications).
E stands for eyes and emotions.
F stands for your foot health.

.

Are there any doctors that specialize in diabetes care?

Yes, there are diabetologist. However I recommend you see a general endocrinologist and who is willing to take care other general conditions.

Diabetes might have other conditions like low T for man, polycystic ovarian syndrome for woman, low libido, UTI, obesity, hypertension, high triglycerides, high cholesterol, etc.

It would be absurd to see a doctor for every single disease. Many other endocrine diseases can also cause diabetes like Cushing's disease and acromegaly. I had a patient who was referred to me for diabetes. It turned out he had another endocrine disease which caused his diabetes.

As I discussed before, strictly speaking, diabetes is not a diagnosis. It is just a sign of high sugar in the blood.Therefore, you will be well taken care of if you choose a general endocrinologist instead of a specialized diabetologist. In my view, a general endocrinologist is better than a doctor who just takes care of "diabetes."

Chapter 6: Diabetic education

When should I get diabetic education?

Diabetes is a very complicated disease. It is not a single standalone disease. It affects every part and every system in your body. New treatments and new ideas are popping up all the time. We are learning and studying to keep up with it every day.

Diabetic education is ongoing. Diabetes is a lifelong disease and you need to learn every day.

What can I learn from diabetic education?

Anything you think might be related to diabetes.

What do I need to do to prepare for one-on-one diabetes education?

You can bring your questions or just be ready to receive some new information from your educator.

What should I do if my doctor and diabetic educator tell me different thing?

You should raise the concern to your doctor to clarify and if confirmed you should listen to your treating doctor.

Chapter 7: How is type 1 diabetes treated?

Questions about curing type 1 diabetes

Can we cure type 1 diabetes with a pancreas transplant?

Progress is being made every day. Successful pancreatic transplants can eliminate the need for insulin injections.

Where can I get an islet transplant or a beta cell transplant?

There are some successful and promising cases for islet transplant or beta cell transplant, but they are still in the research stage. They are not widely available to patients yet. In America, there is a research consortium-CIT.

The Clinical Islet Transplantation (CIT) Consortium is a network of clinical centers and a data coordinating center established in 2004 to conduct studies of islet transplantation in patients with type 1 diabetes.

If you have a strong interest in transplants, you can contact the Consortium members for further information.

http://www.citisletstudy.org/

The network includes the following centers:

University of Miami
Miami, Florida

University of Pennsylvania
Philadelphia, Pennsylvania

Northwestern University
Chicago, Illinois
University of Wisconsin
Madison Wisconsin

Massachusetts General
Hospital
Boston, Massachusetts
Emory University
Atlanta, Georgia
University of Illinois at
Chicago
Chicago, Illinois
Karolinska University
Stockholm, Sweden

University of California
San Francisco, California
University Hospital
Rikshospitalet
Oslo, Norway
University of Minnesota
Minneapolis, Minnesota

University of Alberta
Edmonton, Alberta, Canada
Uppsala University
Uppsala, Sweden

How far away is the artificial pancreas?

It is here. The FDA has already cleared the Medtronic MINIMED
670G system which is the first "artificial pancreas" available to
general type 1 patients. The technology is getting better every day.

Questions about medications, insulin pumps and monitoring

Are there oral medications for type 1 diabetes?

So far, the FDA has not approved any oral diabetic medications for
type 1 diabetes.

Are insulin pumps better than multiple daily injections?

Yes, I recommend an insulin pump to every type 1 diabetes patient if
they can afford it and are able to operate it.

How can I motivate my child to check his or her sugar?

We have technology called CGM. Dexcom is your choice.

Chapter 8. Questions about high and low blood sugar levels, and diabetic emergencies

What is the effect of exercise on blood sugar?

Exercise can increase or decrease your sugar depending on the intensity and time. It is certainly also affected by the food you eat before the exercise.

What symptoms or signs might indicate low sugar?

When sugar is low, your adrenaline is secreted. It causes you to have heart palpitations, sweating, pale skin, shakiness, anxiety, irritability, tingling, anxiety, irritability, and hunger. You might wake up drenched in perspiration and/or crying out during sleep.

As hypoglycemia worsens, you might develop confusion, abnormal behavior or both. You may also experience the inability to concentrate, and difficulty in completing routine tasks. Visual disturbances may occur such as blurred vision. If these are severe enough, they can cause seizures, loss of consciousness, or death.

What should I do if I feel my sugar is low?

You should stop whatever you are doing especially if you are driving. You also need to check your sugar and treat yourself. If you do not know why it happens, see your doctor ASAP.

How should I treat low sugar?

Usually, it is recommended to have 15 grams of carbs and then wait for 15 minutes to make sure your sugar is back to normal.
Here are some examples of 15 grams of carbs:
- Four glucose tablets (four grams per tab)
- One-half cup (4 ounces or 118 ml) of fruit juice
- Four ounces of regular, non-diet soda
- Five hard candies
- One tablespoon (tbsp.) or 15 ml of sugar - plain or dissolved in water
- One tbsp. (15 ml) of honey

If your sugar is not back up over 70 after 15-20 minutes, you need to repeat the process.

I recommend that you always have some glucose tablets in your purse or in your car's glove compartment. Depending on the situation, there are lots of other ways to treat your low sugar. If your sugar is low just before your meal, you can just go ahead and have your meal. Depending on your sugar level, and diabetes regimen, you need to adjust your medications.

When you see your doctor, you need to report this situation.

What do you recommend most for your patient to treat low sugar?

I recommend glucose products (tablets, drinks, powder). When your sugar is low, you want to raise it fast. Glucose products are absorbed fast and this is the sugar your brain can use directly. This will release your symptom faster.

Can you provide some glucose product brands and tell me where to buy them?

For liquids: Relion Glucose Shot, Trueplus Glucose Shot, can be purchased from Walmart. Dex4 can be purchased from CVS.
For powder: Elovate15 can be purchased form Walmart.
For tablets: Relion Glucose tab (4 g per tab), Glucolift glucose tab (4 g per tab) can be purchased from Walmart. Dex4 glucose tab (4 g per tab) can be purchased from CVS. Trueplus glucose tab (4 g per tab) can be purchased from Mejer or Walgreen.
For gels: they come as different grams. I recommend you stick to above three forms.

I eat a lot of stuff, but I still do not feel good. What should I do?

The response to low sugar is the activation of sympathetic nerve system and stress hormones like adrenaline, cortisol. Even your sugar become normal, you need time to metabolize these stress hormones. Therefore, I recommend you eat 15 grams of carbs and wait 15-20 mins and check your sugar again. If still be <70, then you can eat or drink another 15 grams of carbs. If you just based on your feeling, you might eat your refrigerator and still feel your sugar is low. You sugar will rebound to way too high. Remember, you might need to adjust your regimen. Talk to your physician.

What should I do if my sugar is low and I do not feel it?

Here, we assume that you do not have any hypoglycemic signs or symptoms, but your meter shows that you have sugar below 60-70. Here are two scenarios.

Scenario 1: Your sugar is not actually low, but your sugar meter is showing that it is low. In other words, the meter you are using may not be accurate. Occasionally, glucometers can have problems with accuracy.

Based on new FDA regulations, if a patient's blood sugar is below 75, the reading should be within plus or minus 15 of the actual sugar, 95% of the time. For example, if your actual blood sugar is at 70, the meter is acceptable within the new FDA guidelines to show 60. In these situations, you need to make a judgment call. If your sugar is below 60, but close to 60, and if you are feeling fine, and if you are going to eat, you can continue your current regimen.

If you are on a multiple daily insulin shot regimen, you can give half of your premeal insulin before the meal and give the other half of your insulin when you eat or after you eat.

Scenario 2: If you have hypoglycemia unawareness, then you need to be more cautious. You have to treat every low sugar reading as an actual low sugar condition.

What should I do if I cannot feel when my sugar is truly low?

This is called hypoglycemia unawareness, which is very serious and has severe consequences.

Here are the five recommendations I usually give to my patients who have hypoglycemia unawareness.

1. Ask for CGM (continuous glucose monitoring) if your insurance will pay and/or you can afford it. This device can be a lifesaver for patients with hypoglycemia unawareness. For details, please see CGM section.

2. Check your sugar more often, especially before you drive (ideally not driving if possible); check your sugar before and after exercise in addition to before meals and at bedtime.
3. Use an insulin pump that will shut down if your sugar is low.
4. Talk to your family, friends and coworkers to let them know if they notice you are acting weird or having some bizarre behavior, that they need to alert you to check your sugar.
5. Talk to your doctor and he or she will raise your sugar levels, and in most cases, your sense of hypoglycemia will return.
6. Create a higher diabetes control target.

What bizarre behaviors do your friends and family need to pay attention to?

You need to tell your friends, family and coworkers that if you have these symptoms your sugar might be low. Tell them they need to alert you to check your sugar and treat it accordingly.

Here are the seven symptoms to watch for:
1. Irrational thoughts
2. Anger or irritability -- see also Anger During Lows
3. Running away
4. Insisting "I feel fine" in the midst of very unusual behavior
5. High stress
6. High emotions
7. Laughing and silliness

How do I regain hypoglycemia awareness?

Please also see the type 1 diabetes section.
The good news is that you can regain your hypoglycemia awareness by avoiding low sugar. Avoidance of low sugar enables people with diabetes to regain their symptoms when they become low. Here are four things you can do:
1. Set your goal or target to be higher than before. You need to call your doctor and tell him or her what is happening. He or she will carefully adjust your insulin doses or oral medications to closely match your diet and exercise regimen.

2. You should continue to be more alert to physical warnings for 48 hours following a low blood sugar episode.
3. Consider any blood sugar below 60 mg/dl (3.3 mmol) as serious and practice ways to avoid them.
4. Use your records to predict when lows are likely to occur.

What happened when my sugar is not low, but I feel like my sugar is low?

This is a complicated situation. This happens sometimes when your blood sugar has not been controlled for a long time, and then suddenly you take measures to lower your blood sugar. Your body is still used to high sugar, and now they are normal, but your body thinks it is too low. My recommendation is that at that moment you can eat something or treat it as low sugar to ease your symptoms. I recommend you correct your sugar slowly and then your body sense will be back to normal.

I have patients with anxiety which can have similar feeling. If this is the case, certainly you do not need to eat or to increase your sugar if it is normal or high already.

Is CGM the best technology to prevent hypoglycemia?

Yes.

When should I use the glucagon shot my doctor prescribed for me?

This is not for you to use. This is for family members or other bystanders to use to treat your low sugar if you become unconscious and you are not able to eat or drink. Do not use it if your sugar is simply low.

How should I use the glucagon shot?

Educate your family or whoever may be able to help you in emergency situations. Here are three recommendations:
1. After you fill the prescription, open it to review with your family or the people who might be available to help you.

2. Watch a YouTube instructional video together about how to use it and when to use it.
3. If one of your kits has expired, do not throw it away. You can use this kit to practice. Do not inject yourself; inject into a sponge or something safe.

Here are two things to remember about glucagon shots.

1. The injection sites are the same sites as insulin injection sites, like the abdomen, outer shoulder, and outer thigh.
2. Turn the patient to his left or right side since glucagon may cause vomiting.

If you used your glucagon shot, you need to go to the ER and see your physician ASAP to make sure nothing else going on or you might need to adjust your regimen.

Is it true antibiotics like Fluoroquinolones can cause fatal hypoglycemia?

FDA has issued a warning about Fluoroquinolones (Avelox, Cipro, ofloxacin, Levaquin) causing severe hypoglycemia and disturbance in attention, memory impairment and delirium in 2018. Previously. FDA also warned about fluoroquinolone's adverse effects of tendinitis and tendon rupture.

Questions about ketones, high sugar and diabetic ketoacidosis (DKA)

When do I need to check urine ketones?

Ketones are produced when your body does not have enough insulin to use glucose as fuel, so it instead uses your fat stores as fuel. If severe enough, it can cause ketoacidosis which can be life threatening.

Ketoacidosis usually occurs in type 1 diabetes, although it can sometimes occur in type 2 diabetes.

However, in clinic, we usually do not discuss ketones if you have type 2 diabetes and have never had ketoacidosis before. However, be aware many type 1 diabetes are wrongly diagnosed as type 2 diabetes.

Under the following conditions, or any time you think you might have ketoacidosis, please check your urine ketones. You can buy test strips from your local pharmacy without a prescription, although you can also ask your doctor for a prescription.

- You feel sick, especially with nausea, vomiting, or abdominal pain even if you were given the diagnosis of type 2 diabetes when you are on one of SGLT2 antagonist like Invokana, Farxiga, Jardiance or Steglatro.
- You cannot get your sugar under control if you have type 1 diabetes and your sugar are persistently higher than 250.
- If you have fever, >100° F
- If your skin is flushed
- If your breath smells "fruity"
- If you feel like your brain is "foggy"

What do I need to do if my ketones are positive?

You need to call your doctor.

Most likely, you will need to go to ER to make sure you are properly treated, especially if your sugar cannot be controlled. You may have severe dehydration.

What should I do if I have nausea and vomiting and I am unable to keep anything down?

You need to go to the ER.

What should I do if my sugar goes above 500 after a steroid shot?

Steroids are commonly used for many conditions, and they can increase your sugar significantly. It is not uncommon for your sugar to go over 500 after a steroid shot.

Here are the things you can do:

First, you need to make sure you do not have any other sicknesses, such as a cough or a urinary problem. If you feel really badly, go to the ER.

Otherwise, you can try the following:

- Call your doctor or visit your doctor's office for advice.
- Drink plenty of water.

- Cut down on all the carbs you are eating.
- Eat only green vegetables.
- If you are taking insulin already, increase your pre-meal insulin by 20-30% at first and then up to double your dose, and then continue sliding scale (corrections).
- If you cannot get it down, go to the ER or your doctor's office.

What should I do if my sugar goes over 500 and I am not taking steroids?

Do not panic. Calm down and ask yourself if there was anything you ate or did that may have caused the sugar spike. Try to identify the cause and see if the cause can be corrected. If you are fine and your sugar is high, you can try to correct the cause and use the sliding scale to see if you can get the sugar down.

If you have sugar over 500, and you have fever, chest pain, nausea and vomiting, or severe weakness or even confusion, you need to go to the ER.

What are the common reasons for sugar to go over 500?

Based on my patients' reports, the following 10 reasons are common:
1. Steroid use.
2. Common colds, with cold medications. Some antibiotics can cause sugar to spike.
3. Forgetting to take insulin. For type I diabetes, your sugar will go very high if you eat anything with carb and you forget your insulin.
4. Eating or drinking something really sweet. Something with lots of carbs even if it claimed to have "no sugar."
5. Some kind of infection, such as a UTI (urinary tract infection).
6. Alcohol- worse if alcohol is mixed with sugar.
7. Insulin pump problems (insertion cannula kinked, or inserted into a scar).
8. Expired insulin.
9. Dehydration.
10. Stress.

What should I do if for no reason my sugar goes over 500?

You need to go to the ER.

What should I do if my sugar is persistently higher than 250 and I do not feel well?

You need to go to the ER.

My morning sugar is always high. What can I do?

There are a few reasons to have high morning sugar.

- The most common reasons are that you might eat too much at dinner or that you might eat too late at night.
- Snacking is also the common reason.
- Some young people might have "dawn effect" which is caused by morning increased hormones.
- The most important cause is the Somogyi effect which is the rebound from midnight or early morning low sugar.

You should raise this issue to your doctor and identify the cause and treat appropriately.

Chapter 9: How is type 2 diabetes treated?

What is the best medication for type 2 diabetes?

There is no best medication; there is only the most appropriate medication. Your doctor and you should make the decision together.

What is metformin?

Metformin is a biguanide that was first synthesized in 1929 and then clinically developed in the late 1950s by the French physician Jean Sterne, who gave it its first trade name, Glucophage ("glucose eater"). It was introduced as a diabetes medication in 1957 in France and in 1995 in the United States.

What are the brand names for metformin?

Brands: Glumetza, Glucophage, Riomet, and Fortamet

I cannot take the big pill. What can I do?

There are two options for now. You can crush the immediate release form or take the liquid formula. The liquid formula is Riomet. The extended formula should not be crushed.

I cannot tolerate the regular metformin. What options do I have?

Many patients have gastrointestinal side effects, like anorexia, nausea, abdominal discomfort, constipation or diarrhea. Most patients have loose stool, or soft bowel movements, but constipation is also reported by my patients.

I recommend patients take metformin in the middle of the meal. I also recommend my patients to increase the dose slowly. Usually, I recommend my patients start with 500 mg at dinner. After a week, if

tolerated, then add another 500 mg at breakfast. If your maximum daily dose is 2,000 mg after one week, increase the dinner dose to 1,000 mg, and then increase the breakfast dose to 1,000 mg.
Some patients experience a metallic taste in their mouth which can be annoying.

Extended release metformin (metformin ER) is available as generic. You can ask your doctor to switch you to generic metformin ER to try. As a matter of fact, I routinely start with metformin ER.
If your insurance pays, you can also try Glumetza which is the brand name for extended release metformin. Some patients report this is tolerated better.

Does metformin cause vitamin B12 deficiency?

Yes.

Does metformin cause renal failure?

There is no evidence that metformin causes renal failure, but in renal failure patients, I recommend reducing the dose or not using it at all.

Does metformin cause heart failure?

It is still controversial.

Does metformin cause lactic acidosis?

Yes, the good news is that it is very rare if the medication is used appropriately.

When should I temporarily stop metformin?

You should not take metformin if you experience any of the following conditions:
1. You are very sick, with fever, dehydration, especially you have marginal kidney function or history of heart failure;
2. You are not able to drink water or have severe nausea or vomiting;
3. You are going to have a CT scan with contrast, you need to stop and I recommend at least for 2-3 days. If you know that your kidney function is marginal, I recommend you check your kidney function and then restart it.

4. You develop acute kidney failure, you should stop.
5. You develop liver failure, you should stop.

Which oral medication is prone to cause hypoglycemia?

As we know, the sulfonylureas, and glinides will cause hypoglycemia. The glinides are nateglinide (Starlix) and repaglinide (Prandin).

Why are sulfonylureas not so popular now?

Sulfonylureas are not so popular now because the sulfonylureas work by stimulating the pancreas to release more insulin and are only effective when there is some pancreatic beta-cell activity still present.
The most commonly used sulfonylureas are:
- glimepiride (brand name: Amaryl)
- glipizide (brand names: Glucotrol, Glucotrol XL)
- glyburide (brand names: DiaBeta, Glynase PresTab, Micronase).

Hypoglycemia is the most common adverse effect. It can be very dangerous in patients with kidney and liver dysfunction and the elderly. They also cause weight gain.
Furthermore, the long-term effect on cardiovascular outcomes or mortalities is not known and may be adverse.

Why did my doctor switch me from glyburide to glimepiride?

Glyburide has more risk for low sugar.

Should I stop taking sulfonylureas?

If you have other choices, you should stop taking sulfonylureas. Raise this question to your doctor.

Do sulfonylureas cause more heart attacks?

It may be true.

What are DPP-4 inhibitors?

A group of gut hormones was found to be very important in glucose control. They control blood glucose through several mechanisms, including enhancement of glucose-dependent insulin secretion, slowing gastric emptying, and reduction of postprandial glucagon and reduction of food intake.

One of these important gut hormones is GLP-1 (glucagon-like peptide-1). Unfortunately, it is very unstable. The half-life is a few seconds. It turns out GLP-1 is degraded by an enzyme called DPP-4 (dipeptidyl peptidase 4). The group of medication DPP-4 inhibitors inhibits the DPP-4 enzyme, thereby increasing the group of gut hormones like GLP-1.

What are the DDP-4 inhibitors currently on the market?

Current FDA approved DDP-4 inhibitors	
Name	**Active ingredient(s)**
Januvia	sitagliptin
Janumet	sitagliptin and metformin
Janumet XR	sitagliptin and metformin extended release
Steglujan	sitagliptin and ertugliflozin
Onglyza	saxagliptin
Kombiglyze XR	saxagliptin and metformin extended release
Qtern	saxagliptin and dapagliflozin (Farxiga)
Tradjenta	linagliptin
Glyxambi	linagliptin and empagliflozin
Current FDA approved DDP-4 inhibitors-cont'	
Name	**Active ingredient(s)**
Jentadueto	linagliptin and metformin
Jentadueto XR	linagliptin and mefromin extended release
Nesina	alogliptin
Kazano	alogliptin and metformin
Oseni	alogliptin and pioglitazone

What should I know before I begin to take a DPP-4 inhibitor?

Here are seven things you need to know:

1. If you have a personal or family history of pancreatitis, pancreatic neoplasms or cancer, you should not take it.
2. If you have a very weak immune system-easily get all sorts of infection, discuss with your prescribing physician.
3. If you have a history of heart failure, especially active phase, it may not be a good idea to take it.
4. If you have poor renal function, the dose for Nesina, Januvia or Onglyza needs to be adjusted. Tradjenta doses do not need adjustment.
5. It is very rare, but it is reported that this group of medications, like other medication, might cause hypersensitivity, which can be life-threatening.
6. Although uncommon, cases of hepatic dysfunction have been reported in patients taking vildagliptin (I have never use it) and saxaglipitn.
7. DPP-4 inhibitors also have been associated with severe joint pain, especially Januvia and Onglyza. The real connection is not clear.
8. If you are using the DDP-4 inhibitor combinations with metformin, you need to read the metformin section also.
9. If you are using the DPP-4 inhibitor combination with SGLT2 inhibitor, you need to read the SGLT2 inhibitor section also.

I heard that DPP-4 inhibitors cause heart failure. Is it true?

In April 2016, the FDA issued a label change for Onglyza and Nesina. These drugs might be associated with heart failure. It is still not clear if it is agent specific or a class effect.

When should I temporarily stop a DPP4-inhibitor?

If you have any of the following conditions, you should not take any DPP4-inhibitor:
1. You have pancreatitis or a family history of pancreatic cancer.
2. You are very sick with a fever and/or dehydration, especially if you have marginal kidney function or a history of heart failure.

3. You are not able to drink water or have severe nausea or vomiting.
4. You are on a metformin combination, and you are having a CT scan with contrast. Stop taking it 2-3 days before the CT scan. If your kidney function is marginal, I recommend you check your kidney function before you start taking it again.
5. You develop acute kidney failure.
6. You develop liver failure.
7. You are very sick and hospitalized.

What are GLP-1 agonists?

GLP-1 is a gut enzyme which has a series of effects on sugar homeostasis. It enhances glucose-dependent insulin secretion, slows gastric emptying, and reduces postprandial glucagon (glucagon is a hormone which can increase sugar) and helps to reduce food intake. For now, they need to be injected.

What are the currently GLP-1 agonists on the market?

Currently, we have eight products in the US, and more may be in the pipeline.
1. Bydureon BCise (exenatide) - taken once weekly
2. Byetta (exenatide) - taken twice daily. I do not use it any more
3. Trulicity (dulaglutide) - taken once weekly
4. Victoza (liraglutide) - taken once daily
5. Adlyxin (lixisenatide)-take once daily
6. Qzempic (semaglutide)-take once weekly
7. Xultophy (Victoza+Tresiba) in the US and IDegLira in Europe. Tresiba is a long-acting insulin (more details in my <<Diabetes All About insulin>> book.
8. Soliqua 100/33 combines Lantus, a long-acting insulin, with lixisenatide, a GLP-1 agonist, in a once daily shot. I started using it in February 2017. My patients seem to like it better having one shot a day instead of two shots (more details in my <<All About insulin>> book.

How to adjust the dose of Victoza?

I like Victoza. Although it is a once daily agent, it can be adjusted through a wide range of doses. It can be used in a wide range of renal functions. It can be stopped quickly in the case of side effects or if other conditions develop that require it to be stopped. The side effects are usually gone in a day.

I usually instruct patients to start with 0.6 mg 30-60 mins daily before breakfast for one week, if tolerated, move it up to 1.2 mg daily the next week, and then to 1.8 mg daily. The point is to use the maximally tolerated dose. If a patient cannot tolerate 0.6 mg, I instruct the patient to try a smaller dose of 0.12 mg or 0.3 mg. There are no marks for these settings on the pen, but there is a way to do it. Between 0 to 0.6 mg there are 10 clicks. You can count 2 clicks (0.12 mg), you can count 5 clicks (0.3 mg). If you inject one click more or less, do not worry about it.

How to adjust the dose of Ozempic?

Ozempic (semaglutide) is a new member of GLP-1s. It comes with 2 different dosage of pens. One dosage pen can deliver 0.25 mg or 0.5 mg every shot. The other one can deliver 1 mg every shot.

- Start at 0.25 mg once weekly. After 4 weeks, increase the dose to 0.5 mg once weekly. If after at least 4 weeks additional glycemic control is needed, increase to 1 mg once weekly. Usually I give my patients a sample pen first to see what dose he or she needs, and then I give prescription.
- Administer once weekly at any time of day, with or without meals. I recommend you stick to the same day of the week.
- Inject subcutaneously in the abdomen, thigh, or upper arm.

After using Bydureon, I have a small "bump" at the injection side. What should I do?

It is the way by which the medicine is released. Therefore, most time and most people can have a "bump" or "nodule". It usually will go away in 4 weeks. As any other injections, you should rotate your injection side.

If you have injection side reaction, like severe redness, swelling, skin pealing, then you should not continue to take the medication and seek your physician's help.

What should I know before I begin to take GLP-1 agonist?

These are the important things to keep in mind:

1. If you have a personal or family history of pancreatitis, pancreatic neoplasms or cancer, you should not take it.
2. If you have a very weak immune system and easily get all sorts of infections, discuss this with your prescribing physician.
3. If you have a history of heart failure, especially active phase, it may not be a good idea to take it.
4. If you have poor renal function, Adlyxin, Byetta or Bydureon should not be used.
5. It is very rare, but it has been reported that this group of medications, like other medications, might cause hypersensitivity which can be life threatening
6. Family history of a rare thyroid cancer like medullary thyroid cancer or multiple endocrine neoplasia 2A or 2B.
7. GLP-1 agonists slow gastric empty. It might affect other medication absorption. You need to let your doctor know all the medications you are taking. If you are taking some medication which need rapid absorption or need peak concentration to have effect (like some antibiotics), you might not be able to take it.
8. GLP-1 agonists can be put on hold if you are severely sick, for example, if you have a fever, severe nausea, vomiting, and dehydration. Remember, it is okay to hold these drugs on occasions like these.
9. If you have a diagnosis of gastroparesis, you should not take it unless you specifically discuss this with your treating physician.
10. GLP-1 agonists are not insulin, but if you are using them with insulin or sulfonylurea or insulin releasing agents like glipizide, glimepiride or glyburide or glinides like Starlix, they can cause hypoglycemia. Therefore, the dose of insulin or sulfonylureas or glinides might need to be adjusted.

11. As we can see, now we have insulin and GLP-1 agonist combinations. If you are using Soliqua 100/33 or Xultophy, the combination of insulin and GLP-1 agonist, therefore the risk for low sugar is significantly increased.
12. GLP-1 agonists are proteins and might induce antibodies. Although in most cases this does not affect the efficacy or safety parameters, some patients develop high levels of antibodies that may decrease the glycemic response. If you think the effect of your medication is down, talk to your prescribing physician. He or she might be able to change the drug.

What should I do if I have too much nausea when I take a GLP-1 agonist?

Nausea is very common with the use of GLP-1 agonists.

Nausea usually goes away in a week or two. Vomiting is less common. I usually ask patient to stop using it if vomiting occurs. Please read the previous question again.

Always, start with the low dose and then advance to the higher dose. If you are using Victoza, you can reduce to 0.2 and then gradually advance the dose.

If you are using Adlyxin, it takes 2 weeks to advance to next dose. If you are using Ozempic, it takes 4 weeks to advance to next dose.

What is an SGLT2 inhibitor?

SGLT2 is a protein in humans that facilitates glucose reabsorption in the kidney. SGLT2 inhibitors block the reabsorption of glucose in the kidney, increase glucose excretion, and lower blood glucose levels. This is a new class of diabetes medication that can help you lose up to 100 g of sugar in the urine every day.

Which SGLT2 inhibitors are currently on the market?

Here are the 11 medications on the US market, some with metformin or DPP-IV inhibitors:
1. Farxiga (dapagliflozin)

2. XigduoXR, Farxiga (dapagliflozin) with metformin extended release
3. Qtern, Farxiga (dapagliflozin) with Onglyza (saxagliptin)
4. Invokana (canagliflozin)
5. Invokamet, Invokana (canagliflozin)with metformin
6. Jardiance (empagliflozin)
7. Synjardy, Jardiance (empagliflozin)with metformin
8. Glyxambi, Jardiance (empagliflozin) with Tradjenta
9. Steglatro (ertugliflozin)
10. Steglujan, Steglatro (ertugliflozin) and Januvia (sitagliptin)
11. Segluromet, Steglatro (ertugliflozin) and metformin

What should I know before I begin to take SGLT2 inhibitors?

You should know the following information before you take SGLT2 inhibitors:

1. The mechanism of this group of medication is to block the sugar reabsorption, so the sugar is removed in the urine. Just as in poorly controlled type 2 diabetes, the risk for UTIs and yeast infections is increased significantly.
2. Low blood pressure can occur. Loss of sugar also causes loss of water. If you do not drink enough water, you might feel dizziness and low blood pressure. If you are taking a diuretic, then you might need to adjust the dose or stop it. You might also need to adjust other blood pressure medications.
3. Again, if you are dehydrated, you might get an acute kidney injury.
4. In an Invokana clinical trial, the chances for bone fractures were increased. Bone fractures occur more frequently in patients taking canagliflozin (Invokana). I suspect this is caused by low blood pressure which caused the patients to fall. Therefore, it is very important that you drink plenty of water.
5. Patients treated with this group of medications are reported to be more prone to develop diabetic ketoacidosis. This is a serious condition and can be life threatening. The exact mechanism is not known, but normal sugar levels delay the recognition of this condition by both the patient and physician.

6. In an ongoing trial with a mean of 4.5 years of follow-up, there were increases in leg and foot amputations (predominantly toes) in patients taking Invokana (7 versus 3 out of 1000 patients with 100 mg of Invokana and placebo respectively).

7. On Aug. 29, 2018, the Food and Drug Administration (FDA) released a safety announcement warning of a potential link between a rare, destructive bacterial infection – Fournier's gangrene (genital area severe infection) and SGLT2 inhibitors. I do not remember to use on extreme obese patients or for any reason, you can not dry your private area very well.

8. SGLT2 inhibitors can be put on hold if you are severely sick with symptoms of a fever, severe nausea, vomiting or dehydration. Remember, it is okay to put the medicine on hold during these occasions.

What can I do to reduce the chances for UTIs or yeast infections?

UTIs (urinary tract infections) and yeast infections are big issues for women. The chances of having these infections are very high. In clinical trials, they are reported at around 10%. In my experience, I think it is underreported.

Here is what you can do especially if you are a woman:
1. Drink lots of water, always bring water with you wherever you go. Every day, you need to drink at least 64 ounces of water.
2. Have two showers a day (morning and night).
3. Relieve yourself after sex.
4. Wash your private parts well after sex.
5. If possible, have Diflucan handy, when you suspect you have a yeast infection, you can take one. One tab is enough. So, you do not have to wait and suffer. Certainly, you should stop SGLT2 inhibitor for a few days. If you have repeated infection, you should not continue to take it.

Lawyers have Ads on TV, should I stop the medication?

No. Do not let a lawyer be your doctor. Let a doctor be your doctor. Listen to your doctor for medical advice and not a lawyer on TV.

When should I temporarily stop an SGLT2 antagonist?

If you have any of the following conditions, you should not take an SGLT2 antagonist;
1. You are very sick with fever and dehydration, especially if you have marginal kidney function or a history of heart failure.
2. You are not able to drink water or have severe nausea or vomiting.
3. You are on a metformin combination, and you are having a CT scan with contrast. Stop taking it 2-3 days before the CT scan. If your kidney function is marginal, I recommend you check your kidney function before you start taking it again.
4. You have acute kidney injury.
5. You have liver failure.
6. You have a urinary tract infection.
7. You are not able to drink water or if there is no place to go to the restroom.
8. You feel dizziness and your blood pressure is low. Certainly, you need to drink more water. You should then see your doctor for a medication adjustment.
9. You are diagnosed with bladder cancer or have a strong family history of bladder cancer.
10. You are frail or you do not want to lose weight.
11. You are very sick and hospitalized.
12. You have pain in your private area (including genitals)

What is acarbose?

Most carbs you are eating cannot be absorbed directly. They need to be digested. Acarbose is called an alpha-glucosidase inhibitor. It blocks the gastrointestinal enzymes (alpha-glucosidase) that convert complex polysaccharide carbohydrates into monosaccharides that can be absorbed. My patients called it "sugar-blocker".

What are the adverse effects of acarbose?

GI (gastrointestinal) side effects are very common. It is reported that up to 73% of patients have excess flatulence and diarrhea.

How do I reduce the side effects of flatulence and diarrhea?

The only way to do it is to reduce your carb intake. Certainly, you can cut down the dose.

However, if you have some special social event to attend and excessive flatulence is not desirable, it is okay to miss the acarbose dose.

What should I do if I have lots of gas when I take acarbose?

See above. You can reduce the carb intake; you can reduce the medication intake. Sometimes, for important occasions when you are around many people, you can miss the dose.

When should I temporarily stop taking acarbose?

If you have any of the following conditions, you should not take acarbose:

1. You are very sick, with fever and dehydration, especially if you have marginal kidney function or a history of heart failure.
2. You are not able to drink water or have severe nausea or vomiting.
3. You have diarrhea.
4. You are bloated. Stop or reduce the dose.
5. You are on a metformin combination, and you are having a CT scan with contrast. Stop taking it 2-3 days before the CT scan. If your kidney function is marginal, I recommend you to check your kidney function before you start taking it again.
6. You are going to attend a social function and "gas" is not desirable.
7. You develop liver failure.
8. You are very sick and hospitalized.

I have type 2 diabetes, why does my doctor prescribe insulin for me?

Type 2 diabetes in the early stage is mainly caused by insulin resistance. However, at the time type 2 diabetes is diagnosed, it may already be in a later stage where there is more than 50% beta cell loss. Beta cells are the cells in the pancreas that secrete insulin. When the sugar is too high, it is toxic to the beta cells. It causes the remaining cells to die or malfunction. The use of insulin can preserve the remaining beta cells.

What should I know before I start insulin?

Here are several things you need to know before you start insulin:
1. Know the basics about insulin. Insulin is the hormone which is responsible to drive the glucose into cells to be metabolized. It will exert its function even when the sugar is already low.
2. Learning the concept of basal (long-acting) and bolus (fast-acting) insulin.
3. Long-acting-insulin usually works longer than 18 hours. It is taken once or twice a day. It starts to work in 1-2 hours.
4. Short-acting insulin starts to work in 15-30 minutes, and it lasts up to 4-5 hours. However, if you have poor renal function, your insulin might act longer, and you might need to reduce the dose.
5. Do not mistake the long-acting insulin for short-acting insulin and do not mistake short-acting insulin for long-acting insulin.
6. The risk for hypoglycemia is increased.
7. Learn the symptoms and signs for hypoglycemia and what to do if it happens.
8. Learn how to treat and prevent hypoglycemia.
9. Learn how to use the correction scale (sliding scale).
10. Learn the parameters to adjust the insulin dose.
11. Learn how to appropriately store the insulin.
12. Learn how to inject insulin.
13. Learn how to transport insulin.

14. Talk to your family about starting insulin and the risks for hypoglycemia.
15. Teach family members or friends who are living with you about your glucagon emergency kit and how to use it for hypoglycemia.
16. Check your sugar before you drive.
17. I strongly recommend you read my other book <<Diabetes All About Insulin More than 400 Questions From Real Patients>>.

Should I give insulin before the meal or after the meal?

For basal (long-acting, slow-acting) insulin, you can give it at any time, before or after the meal. For once a day, it is better to take at the same time each day. For twice a day, take it 12 hours apart.

For bolus (short-acting, fast-acting) insulin, it is recommended to take it before the meal. However, for some circumstances, we also recommend taking with or after the meal. For example, if you do not have an appetite and do not know how much you are going to eat, it is recommended that you take your insulin immediately after the meal or take it as soon as you know how much food you are going to consume.

Alternatively, for this circumstance described above, it is recommended that you take half of the dose before the meal, and then take half after you are able to finish your meal. If your sugar is below 60-70, and if you do not have any low sugar symptoms, to be safe, we recommend you take your insulin after you start eating. Depending on how low the sugar is, you can reduce your dose by 20-80%.

Should I eat snacks on an insulin regimen?

When you take insulin, especially bolus insulin for your meals, snacks are not recommended. Since, when you snack, your next sugar check will be high since most people do not take insulin for snacks.

Some snacks are okay to eat such as no-carb snacks like cheese (be careful about the fat and calories), or all vegetable snacks, or very low-carb snacks.

If you are snacking with some carbs, and you know how to do the carb count and know the carb ratio, you can give a bolus accordingly.

Your time between meals should not be more than 5 hours during the day. Five hours between meals is too long. You should plan your meals so that you eat four meals a day or three meals and a small snack. Your insulin regimen should be designed according to your meal times.

Chapter 10: All about insulin

What is long-acting insulin?

Long-acting insulin starts in 1-2 hours and lasts at least 8 hours. We also call it basal insulin.
Here are the examples:
- NPH
- Levemir
- Lantus
- Basaglar (biosimilar Lantus)
- Toujeo
- Tresiba

What is fast-acting insulin?

Fast-acting is also known as rapid-acting insulin. It usually starts to act in 10-30 minutes and lasts 1-4 hours. We usually use it before meals or for the sliding scale (correction scale).
Currently these are on the market: Humulin R, Novolin R, Humalog, Novolog, Apidra and Fiasp. The latter four are analogs, and their onset of action is slightly faster than Humulin R or Novolin R. Strictly speaking, Humulin R and Novolin R are not fast-acting, but clinically, we use them as fast-acting. Fiasp is the fastest injectable insulin for now. Inhalable insulin Afrezza is the fastest.

Are there any other types of insulin?

Other types of insulin include:

- Short-acting: all fast-acting insulins are short-acting. When some physicians discuss short-acting insulin, they are referring to Regular (R) Humulin R or Novolin R.

- Intermediate-acting insulin: NPH N.

- In this book, I use short-acting insulin, fast-acting insulin, bolus insulin interchangeably; I use long-acting insulin, slow-acting insulin, basal insulin interchangeably.

- Pre-mixed insulin. Premixed insulins combine specific amounts of intermediate-acting and short-acting/fast-acting insulin in one bottle or insulin pen. 75/25, 70/30 Humulin, Novolin, Humalog, or Novolog.

- Combination of long-acting (basal) insulin and GLP-1 agonist: Soliqua 100/33 is a combination of insulin glargine (Lantus) and the GLP-1 receptor agonist lixisenatide (Adlyxin in the US and Lyxumia in Europe). This can be used only for type 2 diabetes.

- Inhaled insulin. Afrezza is a rapid-acting (short-acting) inhaled insulin indicated to improve glycemic control in adult patients with diabetes mellitus. This was approved by FDA in 2014. It is a premeal insulin to be used on both type 1 and type 2 diabetes. In type 1 diabetes, Afrezza needs to be used with long-acting insulin.

Generic/Brand names for rapid-acting and short-acting insulins

Type of Insulin & Brand Names	Onset	Peak	Duration	Role in Blood Sugar Management
Rapid-Acting/Fast-Acting				
Lispro (Humalog)	15-30 min.	30-90 min	3-5 hours	Rapid-acting insulin covers insulin needs for meals eaten after the injection. This type of insulin is often used with long-acting insulin.
Aspart (Novolog)	15-20 min.	40-50 min.	3-5 hours	
Aspart /Niacinamide (Fiasp)	10-15 min	30-40 min	3-5 hours	
Glulisine (Apidra)	20-30 min.	30-90 min.	1-2½ hours	
Short-Acting				
Regular (R) humulin or novolin	30 min. -1 hour	2-5 hours	5-8 hours	Short-acting insulin covers insulin needs for meals eaten within 30-60 minutes.

Brand names for intermediate-acting and long-acting insulins

Type of Insulin & Brand Names	Onset	Peak	Duration	Role in Blood Sugar Management
Intermediate-Acting				
NPH (N)- Novolin N, Humulin N	1-2 hours	4-12 hours	18-24 hours	Intermediate-acting insulin covers insulin needs for about half the day or overnight. This type of insulin is often combined with a rapid- or short-acting type.
Long-Acting				
Insulin glargine (Lantus)	1-1½ hours	No peak time. Insulin is delivered at a steady level.	20-24 hours	Long-acting insulin covers insulin needs for about one full day. This type is often combined, when needed, with rapid- or short-acting insulin in the regimen but not in the same injection.
Insulin glargine 3X (Toujeo)	1-2 hours	No peak; at steady level	24-36 hours	
Insulin degludec (Tresiba)	1-2 hours	No peak; at steady level	36-48 hours	
Insulin detemir (Levemir)	1-2 hours	6-8 hours	Up to 24 hours	

Brand names for premixed insulins

Type of Insulin & Brand Names	Onset	Peak	Duration	Role in Blood Sugar Management
Pre-Mixed*				
Humulin 70/30	30 min.	2-4 hours	14-24 hours	These products are generally taken two or three times a day before mealtime.
Novolin 70/30	30 min.	2-4 hours	Up to 24 hours	
Novolog 70/30	10-20 min.	1-4 hours	Up to 24 hours	
Humalog 75/25	15 min.	30 min.-2½ hours	16-20 hours	

*Premixed insulins combine specific amounts of intermediate-acting and short-acting/rapid-acting insulin in one bottle or insulin pen. The numbers following the brand name indicate the percentage of each type of insulin.

What should I do if I forget long-acting insulin?

This depends on what you are taking and how often you are taking it.

1. If you are taking Tresiba, you usually are asked to take it once a day in the morning or night. If you forget one dose, you can take it as soon as possible. You can go back to the regular schedule of injections as long as your next regularly scheduled injection is at least 12 hours away. If your regularly scheduled injection is within 12 hours, you can give one shot as soon as possible, then give another shot after 12 hours, then go back to your regular schedule.

2. If you are taking Lantus (biosimilar Basaglar) or Toujeo, you are probably taking it once a day. If you forget one dose, catching up is more complicated. If you have your medication, you can give your medication as soon as possible and then depending on the time for the next scheduled dose

to decide how much you should give for the next scheduled dose. If the next dose is still 12 hours away, I recommend that you take half a dose for the scheduled dose. If your next scheduled dose is less than 12 hours away but more than 8 hours away, you can choose to take a third of your usual dose at the scheduled time. If the next dose is less than 8 hours away, just miss a dose but give the next shot 2 hours earlier than your usual time. Whatever you do, you need to check your sugar and give correction if needed. I have more detailed plan and illustration about dealing with all different scenarios, please read my other diabetes book <<All About Insulin More than 400 Frequently Asked Questions from Real Patients>>.

3. If you are taking Levemir once a day, follow 2 above.

4. If you are taking Levemir or Lantus (or Basaglar) twice a day, you can take a dose as soon as you can. Then, you can push your next dose back by 2 hours, and then your next dose by 1 hour, and then back to your usual schedule. For example, if you give yourself insulin everyday at 9 am and 9 pm and you forget your morning dose until noon, you can give it at noon. Based on the schedule of every 12 hours, your next dose should be midnight, but you need to move 2 hours ahead, which would make it 10 pm. The next day, you can return to your regular schedule of 9 am and 9 pm. If you only forget within 2 hours of your normally scheduled time, you can keep your normal schedule without corrections. If you miss your Levemir or Lantus, and you do not have it, then you may just have to wait until your next dose. If you have fast-acting insulin, you can give fast-acting insulin based on the sliding scale.

5. If you are taking NPH every 12 hours, you can follow the same correction as Levemir.

6. If you are taking pre-mixed insulin, and It is much more complicated, you should be better call your doctor for advice.

What should I do if I accidentally inject fast-acting insulin for long-acting insulin?

Sometimes distinguishing long-acting and short-acting insulin can be confusing. I often get calls about what to do if you mixed up the long-acting and fast-acting insulin.

Here is what you need to do:

1. Do not panic.
2. Depending on your sugar level and insulin sensitivity, your reaction to this mistake is unique.
3. Eat a regular meal and give half of the dose of long-acting insulin. If you have the correct dose and regimen, your sugar should continue to be stable. If you are prone to have low sugar, check your sugar every 2 hours to make sure it is stable.
4. If you are in a situation, in which you do not have a meal to eat, you can miss one dose of long-acting insulin. Check your sugar every 1-2 hours to make sure you are not developing low sugar. If you develop low sugar, treat accordingly.
5. If you are alone and you do not have anything to eat, and you cannot check your sugar, call 911 as soon as possible.

What should I do if I accidentally inject long-acting insulin for fast-acting insulin?

It is slightly more challenging in this case, but there is no need to panic. The chances of you developing low sugar is much lower compared to the mistake of injecting fast-acting for long-acting because the fast-acting dose is usually only one third of a long-acting dose.

This can be very complicated. We have different scenarios. The long-acting can be given in the morning or night. The mistake can occur at any time of the day. I have scenario specific recommendations. Please read my other book <<All about Insulin More than 400 Frequently Asked Questions from Real Patients>>. The following are a few scenarios and recommendations:

1. If this happens during the day, you may just omit the fast-acting for the meal. Your sugar will go up, but that is fine. Then, reduce your fast-acting insulin by half for the day.

Again, your sugar might be high for a day, but it is fine. It is important in this situation to make sure your sugar is not low.

2. If you are prone to have low sugar and your next meal is 5-6 hours away, you might need to check your sugar in 4 hours to make sure your sugar is not low.

3. Check your sugar at midnight to make sure it is not low.

4. If you make the mistake at night, again, just to be safe, omit your fast-acting insulin. Your sugar should go up at bedtime instead of going down, but it is fine to have high sugar for one day.

5. Check your sugar at midnight to make sure it is not going too low. If it is, eat a snack, then reduce your second daytime fast-acting insulin by half. Again, your sugar may go up, but this is safer than going down.

6. If you are trying to get your sugar perfect even in this situation, you can give half or two-thirds of your pre-meal insulin again and continue your long-acting schedule if the next long-acting is normally your next dose. If your next long-acting dose is less than 12 hours away, please reduce it by one-third (the amount you have given already).

What should I do if I accidentally inject myself with long-acting as short-acting and short-acting as long-acting?

Things can happen. There is no need to panic.

Some patients have both long-acting and short-acting insulin shots at the same time in the morning, which is no problem. Normally, the long-acting dose is three times more than the short-acting dose, so you have given yourself three times as much of the short-acting dose and one-third of the normal long-acting dose.

In the morning, your sugar may go down because you have too much short-acting insulin. Therefore, you need to eat more for your breakfast. However, for lunch and dinner, if you give yourself the correct dose, then your pre-meal or midnight sugar may go up. You might need to give more sliding scale.

Check your sugar one more time between the meal and midnight to make sure your sugar is not too low or too high. If you follow this schedule, your sugar may be slightly elevated, which is good in this case. After 24 hours, then go back to your regular schedule.

If you are in this situation, and if you still want to be perfect, you can eat twice as much for the meal and give 2/3 of the long-acting basal insulin again. Continue the insulin regimen as usual. Again, it is very important to check your sugar.

Why is pre-mixed insulin not optimal for type 1 diabetes?

Now we have analog pre-mixed insulin and regular fast-insulin pre-mixed.

For Humalog, we have Humalog mix with NPH 75:25 (NPH 75% and Humalog 25%).

For Novolog mix with NPH70:30 (Novolog 30% and NPH 70%).

For regular fast-insulin, we have NPH mixed with Humulin R or Novolin R 70/30 (70% NPH and 30% of regular insulin).

The benefit of pre-mixed is that it is one shot for both fast- and long-acting insulin. There are analog premix insulin and regular premix insulin. The regular premix insulin is more affordable.

Disadvantages for pre-mixed insulin:
1. The ratio for fast-acting and long-acting is fixed. You cannot change
2. Pre-mixed insulin is not easy to adjust. It is difficult to give slding scale or correction scale.
3. Pre-mixed insulin varies widely and needs to be mixed very well before usage.

Why are some insulins clear and other insulins cloudy?

Any insulin with NPH is cloudy. These are Novolin N, Humulin N, and any pre-mixed insulin.

How should I store insulin?

1. For unused insulin vials or pens, they should be stored in a refrigerator and never frozen. They can be stored until the expiration date on the vials or pens.

2. For a used vial, you can store at room temperature or store it in the refrigerator. Either way, it does not affect its potency. However, if you store it in the refrigerator, it is recommended to allow it to warm up to room temperature before giving the injection. This reduces irritation at the injection site.

3. If you start to use the vial, the storage life ranges from seven days to one month depending on the brand. Please check the product package.

4. For pens, after you start using them, do not put them back into the refrigerator. Keep them at room temperature. The following list details common brand storage life:
   - Humalog 100 or 200 (28 days)
   - Humulin N (14 days)
   - Humalog mix 75/25 (10 days)
   - Humalog mix 50/50 (10 days)
   - Humulin mix 75/25 (10 days)
   - Novolin R (28 days)
   - Novolin N (14 days)
   - Novolin 70/30 (10 days)
   - Novolog (28 days)
   - Toujeo (28 days)
   - Tresiba (8 weeks)
   - Lantus/Basaglar (28 days)

Where can I inject?

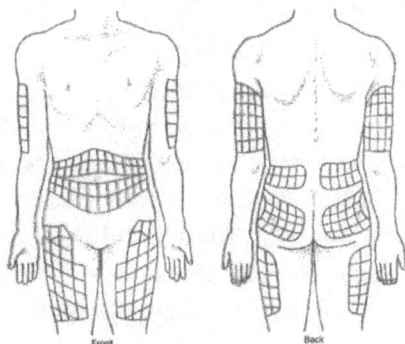

Common insulin injection sites

What else do I need to remember when I do an injection?

1. Only use injection sites that are smooth, with no signs of infection, bumps, or scars.
2. Always rotate the injection site.
3. If you take long-acting insulin, you can inject it on your thigh at night, because you will not be active. Movement and exercise can affect insulin absorption, so you need to be as consistent as possible.
4. Some patients use rotation tattoos, because it helps them keep track of injection sites.

If I have type 2 diabetes. What can I do to prevent weight gain with insulin use?

Insulin is an anabolic hormone, meaning it helps synthesize the building blocks of your body, causing you to gain weight. Most patients on insulin gain weight. But if you take the following measures, you do not need to gain weight.

1. Try not to eat snacks while you are on insulin. Many doctors will ask you to eat snacks to prevent low sugar, but this is wrong. Eating more snacks will cause you to have a higher chance of having low sugar, because when you check your sugar, it will always be high. If your sugar is always high, your doctor will increase your insulin dose because your sugar is not controlled, and you will gain more weight.

2. Try to use the lowest dose possible (for type 2 diabetes). Type 1 diabetes is more complicated. You need to talk to your doctor specifically about this issue.
3. Focus on lifestyle changes.
4. I recommend that you do some sort of exercise before each meal, which will increase your insulin sensitivity, and your need for insulin will decrease.
5. Cut down fat intake. Fat decreases your insulin sensitivity and then your dose will need to be increased.
6. Cut down on carbs. Carbs increases your insulin need.
7. Ask your doctor if you qualify to use insulin in combination with some newer diabetes medications which can help you lose weight. There are the medications: GLP-1 agonists like Byetta, Byduren, Trulicity, Ozempic, Adlyxin, and Victoza; or SGLT2 antagonists like Farxiga, Invokana, Jardiance and Steglatro, as well as their combinations.
8. Ask your doctor to review your medication list to see if you can get off medications that cause weight gain.

Do you have general tips on how to use insulin?

These general insulin shot recommendations are for fixed dose patients.

Maintain a routine of three meals every day and be as consistent as possible with the amount of carbohydrates in each meal. A small snack might be necessary in between meals and at bedtime (see other section for good choices). Exercise helps you burn calories, especially carbohydrates and sugar. A 20-30 minute walk after or before a meal is a good idea! **Keep a written record** of meals, sugar numbers, etc.! You might need to reduce your pre-meal insulin if you plan to exercise before or after the meal (see the exercise section).

Other important tips:
1. Make sure to give yourself short-acting insulin 15-20 minutes before you eat. Fiasp can be given closer to the meal.
2. Check your sugar before you give short-acting insulin. You can adjust your dose based on your sugar numbers. Keep your correcting/sliding scale handy, so you can adjust your insulin doses.

3. Long-acting, Lantus, Basaglar, Toujeo, Levemir, Tresiba is to be injected at the same time every day (usually morning or at bedtime). Tresiba can be injected as a "catch up"—I recommend that you stick to the schedule.

4. ROTATE injection sites as instructed!

5. Physical activity lowers your blood sugar. Check your blood sugar before engaging in strenuous physical activities. Anaerobic exercise will decrease your sugar faster. You need to be more vigilant when you are engaging in anaerobic exercise.

6. You must establish a meal routine (three meals daily) and remain consistent in the amount of carbohydrates as well as controlling your portion sizes. If you would like to eat three meals plus one snack, that is fine. Talk to your doctor, so your regimen can be changed accordingly.

7. Insulin is a treatment, not a cure! DO NOT RELY ON INSULIN ALONE! Healthy eating, physical activity, keeping a record, and testing are the keys.

8. DO NOT STOP injecting insulin without consulting your doctor and/or diabetes educator.

9. Check your sugar before you drive, and always keep some sugar or snacks in your car or purse in case of emergency.

Can you tell me more about basal (long-acting) and bolus (short-acting) regimen?

Usually, you are prescribed two kinds of insulin, long-acting and short-acting. The long-acting insulins (Lantus, Basaglar, Toujeo, Levemir, Tresiba) serve as basal insulin to be taken once or twice a day. Therefore, in discussion, we consider long-acting insulin, basal insulin, and slow-acting insulin interchangeable; we consider short-acting insulin and fast-acting insulin interchangeable.

The basal insulin is used to control fasting and sugar between meals. We usually adjust your basal insulin based on fasting sugar.
The fast-acting insulin (Humalog, Novolog, Apidra, Humulin R, Novolin R and newest member Fiasp) is taken before each meal. This is your bolus insulin. They are for meals. You need to adjust your fast-acting insulin based on your post meal sugar. You can adjust both long-acting and short-acting. Usually, we recommend

adjusting fast-acting insulin (bolus) more than the long-acting insulin (basal).

What is a sliding scale? How do I use it?

The sliding scale is called a correction scale. When you take fast-acting insulin, we usually use the correction scale to correct high sugar. The idea is to get your sugar down by injecting fast-acting insulin based on the scale.

Different patients need different scales. You need to discuss with your doctor what correction scale you need to use. I usually print a scale for my patients.

Please read my other book <<All About Insulin More than 400 Frequently Asked Questions from Real Patients>>. I have very detailed explanation and scales for you to choose from.

I have type 1 diabetes. Do you have general recommendations about how to adjust long-acting insulin?

Life is complicated, and type 1 diabetes and insulin can make your life even more complicated. These are my general recommendations, although you need to speak to your doctor.

1. If you are giving long-acting insulin in the morning, and if your sugar is >80 in the morning, and if you are very healthy and do not get low sugar easily, you can give a full dose of long-acting insulin. If your sugar is below 60, then you might need to eat something first and then give half of the dose. If your sugar is between 60 and 80, you can give half of your long-acting insulin dose. It is important that you need to seek more specific advice from your doctor for your particular situation.

2. If you are giving your long-acting insulin at night, and if your sugar is >130 at bedtime, you can give the full dose. If your sugar is between 100 and130, you might need to cut down your night time long-acting insulin by half or 1/3. If your sugar is below 100, then you might need to eat a small snack and then give a half dose of long-acting insulin.

3. If you have frequently high or low sugar, you need to talk to your doctor. Your insulin regimen might need to be adjusted.

I have type 2 diabetes. Do you have a general recommendation about how to adjust long-acting insulin?

If you are relatively healthy, and if you do not get hypoglycemic easily, you can follow the recommendations I gave for type 1 diabetes above.

If you have multiple comorbidities or are very fragile, I would raise your sugar slightly. If your bedtime sugar is above 160, you can give the full dose. If it is between 130 and 160, you can consider half of the dose. If it is below 130, then you can omit the dose completely.

Chapter 11: Let's talk more about eating

What can I eat?

You can eat anything. Portion control is the key. I have a table to help you choose what to eat in the first part of Chapter 1.

Can I eat fruit? Which ones are the best?

The answer is certainly yes, but you cannot eat too much. Fruits have lots sugar.

Here is the fruit I recommended to my patients the most. Remember, portion control is still very important.

Berries

Blackberries and blueberries are the best. They have low sugar content and might have antioxidants. Raspberries are also very good. The have very low carbohydrates. Cranberries are good, too. Strawberries are not the best, but 3-5 are okay. They can be too sweet.

Goji Berries

I have never seen fresh Goji berries in stores. You can buy them from a Chinese store. They are very low in carbs. In Chinese medicine, they are used to increase sexual vitality. They have lots of antioxidants.

Apples

Most apples are okay for you to have one a day. Eat an apple a day, keep the doctor away! I do not recommend you eat all sorts of fruits in a day. However, Fuji apples are too sweet for you.

Peaches

Some peaches can be too sweet for you. One a day is okay.

Tart cherries

Tart cherries are low in sugar. One cup is fine for you.

Cantaloupe

Some cantaloupe is okay too. One cup is maximum.

Papayas

Papayas are good.

Kiwis, Plums, Apricots and Avocados

These are all good.

When is the best time to eat fruit?

You can eat fruit before or after you exercise.
You can eat fruit immediately after a meal as the dessert if you are on insulin. Your insulin will work on the carbs from the fruit.
If your sugar is not under good control, I do not recommend fruit for you.

What can I eat if my doctor does not recommend fruit for me?

Eat more vegetables instead of fruit. You should eat cucumbers, tomatoes, carrots, mushrooms, cauliflower, broccoli and celery.

Can I snack on fruits?

I do not recommend snacking on fruits. Fruits have too much sugar. It causes your premeal sugar to go up and then your doctor has to increase your diabetes medication. This can be a reason you can not lose weight.

Can I eat sugar-free cookies?

We talked about sugar substitute separately. Sugar-free is not carb free. Cookies may say no added sugar, but they still have many carbs you need to consider.

Can I eat sugar-free ice cream?

Again, sugar-free is not carb free. If you eat one cup, you still have around 30 g of carbs, and 8 g of fat.

Can I eat cheese as snack?

It is true if you eat small amount of cheese as snack, your sugar will not go up. However, most cheese has too much fat or too much salt. If you eat too much, your cholesterol might go up and you might gain weight. If you really want to eat, small portion of reduced fat cheese will be okay.

What are the best vegetables for diabetes?

All non-starchy vegetables are good for diabetes. Here is a list of the most common.

Recommended fresh vegetable list

amaranth greens (Chinese spinach)	greens (collard, kale, mustard, turnip)
artichoke	hearts of palm
artichoke hearts	jicama (Mexican turnips)
asparagus	kohlrabi (German cabbage)
baby corn	leeks
bamboo shoots	mushrooms
beans (green, wax, Italian)	okra
bean sprouts	onions
beets	pea pods
Brussels sprouts	peppers
broccoli	radishes
cabbage	rutabaga
bok choy (Chinese cabbage)	salad greens (chicory, endive, escarole, lettuce, romaine, spinach, arugula, radicchio, watercress)
carrots	sprouts
cauliflower	squash (cushaw, summer, crookneck, spaghetti, zucchini)
celery	sugar snap peas
chayote squash	Swiss chard
coleslaw (packaged, no dressing)	tomatoes
cucumbers	turnips
daikon (Chinese radish)	water chestnuts
eggplant	yard-long beans

Can I drink too much tea?

Well, it is not good to have too much for anything. Too much tea might disturb your sleep because it is a stimulant. Recently I had a patient who drank too much tea and developed renal failure because of that.

What are your favorite foods, and how do you prepare them?

Asparagus

Asparagus is my number one favorite. When I am home alone, this is the one dish I go to. It is so easy to prepare. I sometimes grill, bake, or just pan-fry it. In reality, I do pan-fry more often. I just cut off the dry ends, and then rinse them. I add some vegetable oil in the pan to grease the pan, add a little water, put in the asparagus, put it on the stove and turn on the heat. That is it. After you see the steam coming out of the pan, you just stir a few times until it is dry (do not add too much water—otherwise it will never dry). That is it.

Celery

My second favorite is celery. Most of the time, I just boil it until it soft, and then I add some soy sauce. Sometimes, I cook it with tofu. I boil celery as above and cook my tofu separately. Then I mix them together with some olive oil. You can add some black pepper or any other spices if you like.

Carrots and daikon soup

My third favorite is carrots and daikon soup. American soup is mostly cream based, or broth based. It either has too much salt or too much fat. This soup is good. It does not have fat, and it does not have too much salt. You just cut some daikon and carrots into cubes, add a few dried shrimps (you can buy them from an Asian grocery store), add an appropriate amount of water and boil until soft. You can eat this before your meal to curb your appetite. You can also use it as a snack.

Spinach

Another of my favorites is spinach. I eat it by itself or with bean sprouts. You can eat it raw, but I prefer to stir-fry it with a few drops of vegetable oil.

Zucchini

There is nothing easier than cooking zucchini. You can cut zucchini into whatever shape you like. Just stir and fry. It is also easy to grill.

Chicken broccoli

You might have been to a Chinese restaurant and had chicken broccoli. I usually use chicken breasts which are easy to deal with. I cook the broccoli and chicken breast separately. I just cut the chicken into small pieces. Then, I add some chicken seasoning from Sam's Club with garlic. It just takes a few minutes to cook the chicken breasts. I cut the broccoli into pieces, and just boil them until they are a little soft (not too long, otherwise, it will be too soft). Then, I just mix them. You can add salt if you want.

Onions and mushrooms

I use whatever onions I have and cut them into pieces. I stir and fry the onions until soft. I add the pieces of mushrooms and stir and fry for one or two more minutes.

Okra

I love okra. It is so easy to cook. You can stir fry it with minimal oil, you can just boil it, or you can grill it. You can also bake it to make vegetable chips.

Green beans

They are so easy to prepare, just like okra. You can boil them. I like to stir fry or grill them.

Tomato egg soup

Nothing is easier to cook than this soup. You just cut a tomato, put it into boiled water until it boils again. Then add a beaten egg and stir a few times with a spoon. Add whatever seasoning you like. This soup is good to curb your appetite.

Baked or steamed squash such as acorn squash

Squash like acorn squash have lots of vitamins and fiber. It is very easy to cook. I just cut them into pieces and rinse off the seeds and bake them or steam them. You can season with anything you like. The carbs are low. I use them to replace my carbs from potato, rice or bread.

What are your recommendations for breakfast?

Everybody says that breakfast is very important. I get lots of questions about what to eat for breakfast. Most breakfast foods have too much sugar, too many carbs, and too much fat.
Here are the foods I recommend for breakfast. You can make different combinations if you like:

1. Good fruit and berries, as we discussed in the fruit section. I like blackberries, blueberries, cranberries, strawberries, kiwi, guava, cherries, pears, peaches, cantaloupe—with most of them you still need to practice portion control. Fruit has a lot fructose and they are sugar. You can eat them whole, or you can make smoothies.

2. Greek yogurt. Some versions of Greek yogurt have too much sugar. You need to look at them. On top of the yogurt you can add some chia seeds to add some texture to it. Chia seeds also add extra protein and fiber. You can also try adding some flaxseeds onto your yogurt. Flaxseeds have lots of omega-3 oil and magnesium.

3. Try some beans and lentils to replace animal proteins. There are lots of different ways to prepare beans. They are high in protein and relatively low in carbs. They are good replacements for pure carbs. You can buy or make chickpea hummus to eat with whole wheat bread. Edamame can be consumed at any time of the day.

4. Use whole grains to replace refined carbs. You can try barley or buckwheat. You can just boil them or slow cook them overnight. They have lots of magnesium which might help some people relieve leg cramps. Whole grain rye bread is also a better choice.

5. Oatmeal is often recommended. Overnight oats are a good choice. You can put oats, nuts and some milk in a jar and leave it in the refrigerator overnight. You can eat it in the morning.

6. Oat bran flakes are an alternative if you need a quick and easy breakfast.
7. Some whole grain cereal is acceptable.
8. If you buy bread, you need to make sure you buy 100% whole grain bread and no added sugar or honey.
9. Quinoa is also a good choice. It has good protein and fiber. The only thing you need to do is to boil it. Quinoa pasta is also good for dinner.
10. Small amounts of cheese. If you are not picky, you can try some vegetables with cottage cheese in the morning.
11. Eggs. I usually recommend no more than one egg a day, but you might eat a few egg whites in a day.
12. You can eat all sorts of vegetables in the morning too. Why not? We do not eat it because we are not used to it. I like cooked vegetables.
13. Avocado can be added to your variety.
14. You can incorporate some sunflower seeds, some nuts into your breakfast.

What are some of your ideas about snacks?

Now, you know already that I do not recommend snacks, especially if you are on insulin. I am talking about snacking when your sugar is not low. I divide snacks into three tiers: first tier, second tier and third tier. I prefer first-tier.

What are your first-tier snacks?

I recommend first-tier snacks like vegetables. These are low-carb, low-calorie snacks like broccoli, cucumbers, celery, cauliflower, and tomatoes. I also put carrots in this category. In this tier of snacks, you do not really need to worry about portion control. However, do not use dips.

What are your second-tier snacks?

I put low-carb, low-calorie snacks into this tier like nuts (almonds, walnuts, peanuts, pistachios, hazelnuts, cashews, Brazil nuts, pecans). Seaweed is a low-carb, low-calorie snack, but I put it in this tier due to the fact that if you buy it from an Asian store, it has too much salt and oil. If you prepare it yourself, I would put it in the first tier. Some protein bars can be in this tier. I put protein bars in this tier since they have their own portion control. I do not expect you to eat more than one.

What are your third-tier snacks?

I put moderate-carb snacks with a few calories into this tier. You really need to have portion control. Examples are edamame, pumpkin seeds, and cheese. Some good fruit like blackberries, blueberries, and raspberries are third-tier.

Can I eat popcorn as snacks?

Popcorn is a very popular snack in America. Everybody likes it. It smells good and feels healthy and it is "addictive". I recommend not to eat it. If you really want to eat, do not eat those with butter which has lots fat and even trans-fat (the worst fat). One serving (one cup) home air-popped or stove-top popped corm maybe okay. The problem is that when start to eat, it is not possible to stop since it smells so good and taste so good.

What is the best dressing I can use?

We know that salads are good for you, but there are two pitfalls of which you need to be aware.

1. Do not load your salad with high-fat ingredients like lots of cheese, bacon, and croutons.
2. Do not soak your salad in unhealthy dressings. If you do not pay attention to the amount of fat in the dressing, you can defeat the purpose of eating salads.

So, what are the best salad dressings to use? The fact is that you can use any of your favorite dressings. The key is how much and how you use it.

I recommend you put your salad dressing on the side and only use your fork to dip into it. You can dip it once with each mouthful of salad. Be assured, you can use any dressing you like. You are eating healthy. As every food, portion control is always the key.

If you are one of those people who always like plenty of choices, you can choose any dressing. Just limit yourself to two tablespoons.

Just be sure the calories are less than 50 and the salt is less than 300 mg.

How many carbohydrates may I eat?

I recommend a low-carb diet. A very low-carb diet is typically taking 50 grams per day. However, I do not recommend carbs just on face value. Not all carbs are the same, and the food you eat with the carbs also makes a difference to your blood sugar. It is not just how many carbs you eat, it is the kind of carbs you eat, and the other kinds of food you eat with them.

I recommend no refined and processed carbs like white rice and white bread. If these are the only carbs you have, I recommend you eat lots of vegetables first and then eat these carbs. Vegetables are low in carbs and high in fiber. There are no limits on the amount of vegetables you can eat. Beans are high in carbs, but their effect on blood sugar is much less profound. You still need to practice portion control on beans.

Should I calculate my calories every day?

There are ways to calculate the calories. I see a lot of apps that can calculate daily calories for you. However, in the long term, these calculations do not work. The reason is that life is more complicated than calculations. We just eat what we have, and we cannot calculate first and then eat. Moreover, those calculations are not accurate anyway. Our body can adjust our expenditures along with the calorie intake.

What is the best diet?

Read my Obesity Book. Go to Amazon.com and search my name.

People say fiber is good for diabetes. How much fiber should I consume every day?

Fiber is good. Studies show that enough fiber actually reduces the postprandial sugar. It also lowers the risk of cancer, lowers blood pressure, lowers blood cholesterol and lowers the risk of cardiovascular disease.

Again, I do not recommend that you count your fiber. If you follow the plant-based diet I recommend, you will get more than you need.

My potassium is low. What food is good for me?

I recommend that you take a potassium supplement instead of thinking of getting more potassium from food since in diabetes one of the treatments is to control your food intake. However, you might be able to incorporate the following food into your diet.

1. **Nuts:** Almonds
2. **Fruit:** blackberries, apricots, avocados, dried apricots, bananas, dates, grapefruits, nectarines and oranges.
3. **Vegetables:** broccoli, Brussel sprouts, artichokes, acorn squash, spinach, mushrooms, carrots and tomatoes.
4. **Other:** sweet potatoes, coconut water, yogurt, white beans, beets, clams, lentils, okra, soymilk, salmon and tuna.

Chapter 12: Let's talk about sweeteners

What are the Sweeteners?

We know too much sugar is not a good thing. Now people are turning to sweeteners and think they are better alternatives. They may not be.

In the United States, six intensely sweet sugar substitutes have been approved for use. They are stevia, aspartame, sucralose, neotame, acesulfame potassium, and saccharin.

FDA and GRAS approved artificial sweeteners and brands			
Sweetener	**Approval Date**	**Sweetness Factor (Relative to sugar)**	**Products**
Saccharin	1958	200-700	Sweet'N Low, Sweet Twin, Sugar Twin
Aspartame	1981	200	NutraSweet, Equal
Acesulfame Potassium	1988	200	Sunnet, Sweet One
Sucralose	1998	600	Splenda
Neotame	2002	8000	Newtame
Advantame	2014	20,000	
Stevia/rebaudioside			Sweet Leaf, Sun Crystals, Stevia, Truvia, PureVia
Extracts from swingle fruit/monk fruit			

What sweeteners do you recommend?

I recommend stevia and monk fruit extract.

What is stevia?

Stevia is a genus of about 240 species of herbs and shrubs in the sunflower family. These plants are native to subtropical and tropical regions from western North America to South America. The species Stevia Rebaudiana, commonly known as sweet leaf, sugar leaf, or simply stevia, is widely grown for its sweet leaves. In 1931, two French chemists isolated the glycosides that give stevia its sweet taste. These compounds, stevioside and rebaudioside A, are 250–300 times as sweet as sucrose and are heat-stable, pH-stable, and not fermentable.

Truvia is a consumer brand of stevia sweetener contains erythritol and rebiana, marketed by Coca Cola and Cargill.

PureVia is another brand of stevia marketed by Pepsico and Pure Circle.

SweetLeaf is a stevia product by Wisdom Natural Brands
In its history, there has been lots of controversy about stevia's health effects. This includes the possibility it may be carcinogenic. However, it seems safe to say, that when consumed in reasonable amounts, stevia may be an exceptional natural plant-based sugar substitute.
Stevia is now present in a number of foods and beverages in the US, including Gatorade's G2, Vitaminwater Zero, SoBe Lifewater Zero, Crystal Light and Sprite Green.

Where can I buy monk fruit extract?

You can buy from Walmart and other grocery stores.

Can I eat honey or use honey as sweetener?

Honey is actually simple sugar digested by bees. So, it is the same as sugar. I do not recommend using honey as a sweetener.

Chapter 13: Diabetes and exercise

I have type 2 diabetes, and otherwise I am healthy and fit. Is there anything I need to do before I exercise?

If you have type 2 diabetes and no other complications, and if you are not using insulin or some medications like sulfonylureas, which can cause hypoglycemia, you do not have to take diabetes specific precautions. Follow the recommendations for people without diabetes.

If you are taking insulin or medications like sulfonylureas, you might need to reduce medications since exercise might cause hypoglycemia. You also need to exercise with someone in case you develop hypoglycemia and you need to keep a "diabetes kit" with you. In the kit, you need to have a glucometer to check your sugar and some candy or something with sugar, which can raise your blood sugar quickly. If you are taking SGLT2 antagonist like Invokana, Farxiga, or Jardiance or combinations, you need to take extra caution to avoid dehydration. Never exercise without taking water with you.

Can I drink Gatorade or another sport drink while I am exercising?

If you are doing very strenuous exercise like a marathon, then sport drinks might help you. Otherwise, you do not need it.

Do you recommend other sport drinks?

I think most of them are pretty much the same. They do have some difference in electrolytes contents and sugar content. You need to choose a sport drink based on how your body responds to it.
Here is a comparison of some of the popular sports drinks.

Product Serving Size 8 Oz. (240mL)	Total Calories	Total Carbs (g)	Sugar (g)	Sodium (mg)	Potassium (mg)
Accelerade	80	15	14	120	15
CamelBak Elixir	<5	<1	—	136	23
Cliff Shot Electrolyte	80	19	10	180-200	50
Cliff Quench	45	11	10	130	35
Cytomax	71	18	10	96	48
First Endurance EPS	63	16	11	180	107
Gatorade	50	14	14	110	30
Gatorade Endurance	50	14	14	200	90
Gatorade G2	25	7	7	110	30
GU Electrolyte Brew	50	13	4	125	20
GU_2O	<54	13	3	122	21
Heed	51	13	1	20	8
HYPR Sports Drink	71	19	—	151	—
Nuun	<5	<1	—	187	51
PowerADE	60	15	15	52	32
PowerADE Zero	0	0	0	100	250
Propel	10	2	2	75	0
CarboPro 2.6 Oz	200	50	0	150	100

counts your activity. The study also found that the devices were less accurate when worn on the person's dominant wrist.

Should I join a gym?

Studies show people tend to be more active when they join a gym. When you have a paid membership, you tend to exercise more. At the gym, you can also get consults from exercise professionals about what kind of exercise is good for you based on your fitness and physical condition.

I am too busy to do any exercise. What can I do?

Researchers found that short-burst exercise is as good as long and moderate exercise. If you are generally healthy, except for diabetes, you can try some so-called short-burst exercises. Be sure to include at least two minutes to warm up and three minutes to cool down. You can do two minutes of full-intensity exercise such as running or cycling.

When is it better to exercise, before a meal or after a meal?

Studies have found that if you exercise after a meal, your need for insulin will be reduced. When you exercise before a meal, your insulin sensitivity will increase after the meal. If you are taking insulin, you can reduce your insulin use. If you are taking a sulfonylurea medication, you can reduce it also.
My recommendation is that if you are on insulin and your sugar is under perfect control, and if you start walking before or after the meal, you can reduce your insulin by 20% to start with. Based on your response, you can adjust your premeal insulin.

Is it better to exercise after a meal so I will not have hypoglycemia?

It is true your chances of having hypoglycemia are reduced if you exercise after a meal. I do not recommend for you to do strenuous exercise immediately after a meal. However, it is okay to start walking 10-15 minutes after a meal.

I do not have time during the day. Can I do my exercise at night?

This is a difficult question. Exercise has different effects on different people. For most people exercise will increase their alertness due to the secretion of adrenaline and cortisol. These hormones might affect your sleep. If you want to do exercise at night, I recommend you do it two hours before you go to bed. This will minimize the unfavorable effect on your sleep.

What kind of exercise is good for diabetes?

All kinds of physical activities are good for diabetes. Based on ADA research, the two most important types of exercise for diabetes are aerobic exercise and strength training.

What is aerobic exercise?

Aerobic simply means that your cardiovascular system can supply enough oxygen to the muscles for energy. In the gym, it is known as cardio.

Examples of aerobic exercises are:

- cardio machines
- cycling / running
- swimming
- walking
- hiking
- kickboxing
- dancing
- cross country skiing

However, when you perform an exercise at an intensity which exceeds your heart and lung capacity to supply enough oxygen to your muscles, then the aerobic exercise becomes an anaerobic exercise.

What is resistance training?

Resistance training is using weights to train your muscles.
Examples of resistance training are:

1. Using your own body weight--like pushups, pull-ups, abdominal crunches and leg squats.
2. Using free weights, like barbells and dumbbells.
3. Using weight machines. There are many different weight machines you can use if you go to a gym or fitness center. You certainly can also buy a weight machine.
4. Using resistance bands. They come in different strengths and colors. They all are very affordable. You can use them almost anywhere.

I have a history of cardiovascular disease. What should I pay more attention to while exercising?

Here are seven things to pay attention to while exercising:
1. Start slow and increase intensity slowly.
2. Stop if you have chest pain, shortness of breath, or other discomfort. See your cardiologist.
3. Do not get dehydrated.
4. Do not do strenuous exercise under the sun.
5. Do not do exercise under extreme weather conditions.
6. You can do resistance exercises, with low weights and moderate intensity. Do not exceed your capacity.
7. Ideally, get an exercise prescription for a physical therapist.

I have retinopathy. What should I pay more attention to while I exercise?

There are actually different kinds of retinopathy. If you have diabetic proliferation retinopathy, you certainly should not do strenuous exercise or resistance training, since in proliferative retinopathy, the new fragile cells developed on the optic disc. Too much pressure can cause leakage or hemorrhaging into the eye resulting in loss of vision. You may also be at risk for retina detachment.
Therefore, it is recommended that you start slow and go slowly with low to moderate intensity. This includes activities like slow biking, walking, ballroom dancing, and other low-impact activities. Do not do anything with movement that causes you to lower your head or hold your breath.

I have neuropathy. What should I remember when I do my exercise?

Mild neuropathy does not affect your balance, but severe neuropathy does. If you feel unstable, you need to choose exercises that will not cause you to fall.
If your neuropathy does not affect your walking or jogging, it is okay to continue. If your neuropathy is so severe that you are not balanced, you should not walk as an exercise. If you can swim, it is a great exercise. Stationary biking is safe for patients with neuropathy.

Examine your feet before you start exercising and after you finish to make sure you do not have any cuts or ulcers.

I have Charcot foot. What can I do for exercise?

This bad form of neuropathy most often occurs with type 1 diabetes. The foot bones are repeatedly fractured and this causes deformation. You should not walk as an exercise. You certainly should not jog or run. Walking in the pool may be okay depending on your severity. The idea is that you should stay off your feet as long as possible. You should also have diabetic shoes that have a good fit and great support.
Arm biking can be a good form of exercise. Floor exercises are good, too.
If you have access to a pool, swimming will be the best exercise for you. If you do not know how to swim, you can learn or just walk in the pool.
You should not do water exercise if you have an open wound. As a rule of thumb, you should avoid putting weight on your foot when you exercise.
You should exercise with someone else since you most likely have type 1 diabetes which is prone to cause hypoglycemia.

I have nephropathy. What should I pay attention to during exercise?

Strenuous exercise increases your blood pressure and increases your blood pressure to the kidneys. This can increase the protein in the urine and might worsen your nephropathy. Therefore, you should not do strenuous exercise. Chinese Tai Chi is good. Swimming (water aerobics), cycling and Yoga are good, too.

How should I work with a personal trainer?

If you are lucky enough and able to hire a personal trainer, here are some recommendations:
   1. If possible, get a recommendation from your friends who have used the personal trainer before.
   2. Check credentials. Your trainer might be certified under ACSM (American College of Sports Medicine); NASM (National Academy of Sports Medicine); NSCA (National Strength and Conditioning Association).

3. Ask your trainer some questions to get to know them better. You can ask about his or her previous experience working with diabetics and other specific conditions you might have. It is very important to know if he or she has some basic knowledge of diabetes.

4. Write down the list of conditions you have and communicate this to your personal trainer. This is very important. Since certain conditions mean you need to stay away from certain types of exercise. For example, if you have retinopathy, you should not do any exercise to increase the pressure to your retina. If you are not very clear about your condition, you can ask your doctor to help you.

5. Educate your trainer. Let your trainer know how to observe hypo or hyperglycemia and discuss plans to handle problems beforehand.

6. If you have a CGM and insulin pump, educate your trainer about what it can do and what it cannot do.

Chapter 14: Diabetes and travel

What and how should I prepare for my travel?

As we already discussed, there are some general rules, and some specifics you need to consider. Your travel preparations depend on what kind of diabetes you have, what regimen you are on and how you will be traveling. There are many specifics, and we cannot know every scenario, but we will discuss some specifics in the questions that follow.

I have type 1 diabetes and I am using an insulin pump, how should I prepare for travel? Do you have a checklist?

Yes, I do. Here is the checklist for you.
- ✓ Bring your pump. This is obvious.
- ✓ Travel bag.
- ✓ Insulin. Take more than you estimate you might need.
- ✓ Infusion sets. Take more than you need.
- ✓ Batteries. Take extra batteries in the right sizes.
- ✓ Glucometer, strips, lancets and alcohol swipes.
- ✓ Ketostix
- ✓ Your insulin pump failure supplies like insulin pen, needles or syringes
- ✓ Always wear you diabetes alert bracelet.
- ✓ Hypoglycemia kit. Snacks for mild hypoglycemia and your glucagon emergency kit.
- ✓ Do not forget other medications for other conditions.
- ✓ Some antibiotics for UTI or yeast infection if you think you need them.
- ✓ Do not forget your doctor's office telephone number and your pump manufacturer's representative number.

I have type 1 diabetes and I am on basal and bolus regimen. How should I prepare for travel? Do you have a checklist?

Here is a checklist for you:
- ✓ Your insulins both-long-acting and short-acting.
- ✓ Glucometer, strips and lancets and alcohol swipes.
- ✓ Hypoglycemia kit with snacks for mild hypoglycemia and a glucagon emergency kit.
- ✓ Ketostix.
- ✓ Diabetic alert bracelet.
- ✓ Do not forget other medications for other conditions.
- ✓ Some antibiotics for UTI or yeast infection if you think you need them.
- ✓ Do not forget your doctor's office telephone number.
- ✓ Travel bag.
- ✓ Sharps disposal container or similar hard surface disposal container.

I have type 2 diabetes and I am taking insulin. What should I do to prepare for travel?

You should use the checklist above for type 1 diabetes basal and bolus regimen.

I am traveling by plane. Any TSA tips?

Here are some TSA tips for you.
1. Make sure you bring all your medications in carry-ons.
2. Put all the insulin vials and pens in a bag and declare them.
3. You do not need a letter from your doctor to bring diabetes supplies onto a plane. If you want one, you can always ask for one from your doctor's office.
4. If you wear an insulin pump, the pump manufacturer usually advises against it being screened by imaging technology. Technically speaking, there should be no problem for it to be screened by an x-ray or a metal detector. I have patients who say they let their pump go through the x-ray machine. If you don't want to do this, you can let the TSA do a pat down check, then they will usually check for explosive residues.

5. If you wear a sensor, you are advised not to use the whole-body scanner. I do not know of any research, but the manufacturer usually advises against it.

6. If you have further questions or concerns, you can call TSA toll free 855-782-2227.

I have type 1 diabetes, and I am on an insulin pump. I will fly over a few time zones. How do I change my pump settings?

First, as we discussed, you should know your basal rates. Some patients have one single basal rate. Some patients have multiple basal rates and have significant changes. Again, you should be mindful that your basal rate needs changing if your lifestyle changes. Travel changes your lifestyle. Checking your sugar is the key.

Here is a way you can test to see if your basal rate has not changed too much when you get up and when you go to sleep. You can simply keep the same setting and switch to the local time when you get there. You can try the average basal rate as your temporary rate (=total basal units/24), if you have a variable basal rate.

You can also visit your doctor's office. Discuss possible lifestyle changes, and your doctor can set up a second basal rate for you. When you get to the new time zone, you can change the time and restart the basal.

Travel sometimes can be unpredictable. Ask your doctor to recommend a single basal rate based on your proposed activities. Do this if you would like to have a relatively conservative basal rate, and then if your sugar is too high, you can compensate with bolus. Therefore, checking your sugar is the key. Bring more strips and lancets to monitor your sugar since you might test many more times than usual.

I am on long-acting and short-acting insulin. I will fly east over a few time zones. What should I do?

If you fly east, the day of flying will be shorter. If the time change is just under 4 hours difference, you might just reduce your basal by 10-20%, or no change at all if your sugar has not been well-controlled. When you reach your destination, change your watch to the local time and continue your regular basal. You should continue your same bolus dosage, using the insulin carbohydrate ratio and sliding scale (correction).

If you fly east and the time change is 4-8 hours, you can reduce your basal insulin by30% on the day of flying.
If you fly east and the time zone change is over 8 hours, you can reduce your basal insulin by 50%. If you give yourself basal every 12 hours, you can simply miss one dose.

I am on long-acting and short-acting insulin. I will fly west over a few time zones. What should I do to my basal insulin?

If you fly west, the day of flying will be longer. Again, if the time change is less than 8 hours, you might not need to make any changes to your basal insulin. You might just check your sugar 1-2 more times and give some correction if needed.
If you fly west and the time change is 8 hours or more, I recommend you keep your original time zone on the airplane, and give the basal insulin at the usual time. When you get to your destination, you can miss one dose, just use the correction or sliding scale every 4 hours, until the next usual basal dose based on the new destination time. However, if you are using the basal every 12 hours, then you can switch to local time without too much difficulty. You do not need to miss any doses.

I am on oral diabetes medications. What should I do if I travel over a few time zones?

There are a few oral medication categories.
If you are taking sulfonylurea and traveling east, you might want to reduce the dose in the day of travel, or after adjusting to the local time. If you travel to the west and the time difference is less than 8 hours, you can adjust to the local time after your arrival.
If you are taking medications like glinides, you can continue to take it with meals.
If you are taking other medications, you can follow the instructions for sulfonylurea.
If you are taking daily injections like Victoza, it is okay to continue the current regimen with no change. Or, you can miss one dose based on which way you are traveling.
If you are taking a once a week injection, then you really do not need to worry. After arriving in the new time zone, you can continue your regimen.

Chapter 15: How should I prepare for a colonoscopy or outpatient surgery?

What should I do when I am preparing for a colonoscopy?

Colonoscopy is a common procedure that most patients will have at least once in their lifetime. The day before the procedure, you will prepare for the procedure by taking a clear liquid diet and some laxatives.

Diabetes control relies on diet, while medication is adjusted based on your diet. Because your diet is being changed drastically for the procedure, your diabetes medication will also need to be adjusted. Here are some suggestions but you will need to go through these with your gastroenterologist and the doctor who is taking care of your diabetes.

Your diet will be clear liquids.

The following drinks are recommended:

- water (plain, carbonated or fruit flavor)
- fruit juices without pulp, such as apple, or white grape (not red grape juice)
- sodas are fine
- gelatin (no red color)
- tea or coffee without cream or milk
- strained tomato or vegetable juice (not smoothies)
- sport drinks like Gatorade
- clear, fat-free broth (bouillon or consommé-you can buy or make yourself)
- ice pops without milk, bits of fruits

Your medication also depends on how many carbs (sugar) you are drinking. Generally speaking:

- If you have type 2 diabetes and are on oral medications–take half of your medication the day before and do not take any oral medication on the day of the procedure. If you finish the procedure very early in the morning, and resume your diet, you can resume your oral medication.

- If you have type 2 diabetes and are only on metformin, it is okay not to take metformin the day before and on the day you have procedure.
- If you have type 2 diabetes and are on long-acting insulin, you can take half the dose you are taking the day before and on the day of procedure if you have reasonably good control before the procedure. However, if your blood sugar has been over 200, you can continue your usual dose.
- Certainly you need to check your sugar at least 4 times a day, every 4-6 hours and anytime you feel your sugar may be low.
- If you are taking multiple shots, to be safe, I recommend you take ⅓ to half of your dose before each meal(your liquid meal) of the fast-acting and take half of the long-acting. You can continue to use the sliding scale.
- However, if you have type 1 diabetes and you are on an insulin pump, I recommend that you use the half dose on the sliding scale at bedtime. If your blood sugar is reasonably controlled, then you should be able to continue to use your pump the day before. Some gastroenterologists do not feel comfortable allowing you to keep the insulin pump on. If this is the case, it is okay for you to take it off, because most colonoscopies only last 30-60 minutes. However, if you are having a more complicated procedure that you expect to be longer, you need to be on an insulin pump or substitute with basal long-acting insulin.
- If you have type 1 diabetes and you are on multiple shots daily, certainly, you do not need premeal insulin on the day of the procedure since you are not eating. You need to continue the basal insulin and the sliding scale. If you are drinking anything with carbs, you need to give insulin depending on your carb ratio. If you do not know your carb ratio and cannot reach your doctor, you can try to give a third of your fixed dose pre-meal insulin for every cup of sugary drink.

What should I do if I am going to have surgery tomorrow?

For hospitalized surgery, your surgeon or other health care personnel will decide what to do. In the case of outpatient surgery and your surgeon does not give you instructions, here are your guidelines.

Following your surgeon's instructions is very important. These recommendations are not meant to replace your surgeon's recommendations.

This also depends on what type of diabetes, what kind of surgery, and how long your surgery lasts.

1. If you have type 2 diabetes and are on oral medications, if your surgery is minor and your surgeon does not ask you to fast, you can continue your same regimen.

2. If you have type 2 diabetes and are on oral medications, if your surgeon asks you to fast overnight, the second day you can omit the oral diabetes medication. Your surgery team will give you insulin if your sugar is too high.

3. If you have type 2 diabetes and you have gastroparesis, you might want to fast longer than overnight if fasting is required for your surgery.

4. If you have type 2 diabetes and you are on basal insulin, and if your sugar has been well-controlled with no significant lows or highs, no matter what kind of surgery, you can continue the same dose of long-acting basal insulin. If you have had frequent low sugar before, I recommend you to use half of your basal insulin.

5. If you have type 2 diabetes and you are on multiple shots involving long-acting and short-acting insulin, you can keep the same dose of basal insulin, and stop the short-acting dose. However, if you have some low sugar episodes before the surgery, I recommend you to cut down your basal insulin by half.

6. If you have type 1 diabetes, and you are on an insulin pump, and you do not have frequent lows, I recommend keeping the insulin pump on if possible.

7. If your procedure is under 1 hour, it is okay to be off your insulin pump if your surgeon requests. If you expect your procedure to be longer or other things happen, you need to be on basal insulin or fast-acting insulin. Your surgeon should know how to take care of it.

8. If you have type 1 diabetes and you are on basal and bolus regimen, and you do not have significant lows, you can continue to take the same dose of basal insulin. If you

have frequent lows, I recommend you to reduce your basal insulin by half.

9. If you have type 1 diabetes and you are on premix insulin, it can be very challenging. If your surgery is less than 8 hours after your last dose and the surgery is very short, it is okay to miss one dose. If your surgery is longer than 8 hours after your last insulin dose, you need to give yourself some insulin. Discuss this with your doctor beforehand. I recommend you have surgery early in the day so you do not have to fast very long. If you do not have insulin for longer than 12 hours, you might develop DKA (diabetic ketoacidosis).

Chapter 16: Diabetes and gastroparesis

My doctor said I have diabetic gastroparesis. What is it?

The stomach does a lot of work after we eat something. The stomach muscles aided by acid grind food into tiny, tiny pieces. The stomach muscle grinding is initiated by pacer and spread controlled by an internal nervous system. Usually, when eating a balanced meal, our stomachs will empty 60% of the food in 2 hours and empty completely in 4 hours. But if your stomach delays emptying and causes severe nausea, vomiting, early satiety, bloating and or upper abdominal pain, and then we say you might have gastroparesis

Is there anything I need to know before my doctor gives me a diagnosis of gastroparesis?

First, before you go to have your stomach emptying test, you need to get your sugar under control. Since high sugar slows down your stomach, your sugar needs to be under 250 mg/dl on the day of testing.
Second, make sure you talk to your GI doctor about the medications you are taking which might cause gastroparesis.

Which medications can slow down gastric emptying?

In the diabetes world, metformin is the most common diabetes medication. Metformin can slow down gastric emptying and cause you to have nausea and vomiting. You might ask your doctor to see if you can stop taking it for a while.
The second most common medications that slow down gastric emptying are the GLP-1 agonists:
- Byetta
- Bydureon
- Trulicity
- Ozempic
- Adlyxin
- Combinations like Soliqua 100/33 or Xultophy.

93

More medications might come out. So, ask about those. For type 1 diabetes, Symlin (Amylin analogues) can also cause gastroparesis. All these drugs should be stopped.

Are there any medications other than diabetes medications that can delay gastric emptying?

Yes, there are many medications that can delay gastric emptying. This is why you need to talk to your doctor, including your GI doctor, to see if you can quit taking some of these medications. Commonly used medications which can delay gastric emptying are:

- Blood pressure medications like alpha-2 adrenergic agonist like clonidine; calcium channel blockers like amlodipine, Cardene, nifedipine, cardizem.
- Tricyclic antidepressants- luckily these days, we do not use so often, like amitriptyline.
- Some medications, ironically, are used for abdominal pain, like hyoscyamine (Levbid), dicyclomine, Librax, and so on.

Are there any other medical conditions that can mimic gastroparesis?

Some other conditions might mimic gastroparesis. Such as,

- Some psychiatric diseases like depression, anxiety, anorexia nervosa, anorexia bulimia, psychogenic vomiting. Your doctor may have trouble differentiating them. You need to talk to your doctor about everything.
- Functional dyspepsia, which also has early satiety, postprandial fullness, and epigastric pain or burning. This condition can also have slow gastric emptying. Your GI doctor will figure it out for you.
- Cyclic vomiting syndrome. This is another difficult condition to treat and to differentiate. Patients suffering from this condition are characterized by episodes of intense nausea and vomiting lasting hours to days. These are separated by symptom-free periods of variable lengths.

Is there anything can I do to mitigate the symptoms?

Yes, you can do a lot. Here are some of my recommendations:

1. Focus on controlling your diabetes. Check your sugar and take your medicines as prescribed.

2. Do not drink any ice-cold water. The right temperature is important for your stomach to work. Many people are surprised that their stomach works much better after they begin to drink warm water. Think about it. If your stomach has been frozen, how can it move and perform its job of grinding?

3. Cook your food longer. Get a slow cooker. The more thoroughly you cook your food, the less your stomach needs to work. Even if you have severe gastroparesis, your stomach usually does not have trouble handling liquid.

4. Do not eat raw vegetables.

5. Invest in a good high-powered blender like Ninja. Let the machine do more work, and let your stomach do less work.

6. Ask your doctor to review all your medications to see if any of them can worsen your gastroparesis. For the medications which can cause or worsen gastroparesis, please see above.

7. Never ever eat pizza, chicken nuggets, or other high fat foods, especially high animal fat foods like red meat.

8. Do not drink sodas, lemon juice, or orange juice.

9. Do not eat high acidic foods like oranges, or food that is too spicy.

10. Do not eat too much at one meal. Never go to a buffet.

11. Try not to drink alcohol.

12. Certainly, no smoking. Smoking will slow down your stomach emptying. Some patients gain weight after they stop smoking. Stopping smoking is part of the reason they eat more.

13. Jogging and walking actually increase gastric motility. Always take a walk after a meal, but walk slowly.

Do I need to take extra vitamins for gastroparesis?

Yes, I recommend you to take sublingual vitamin B12, vitamin B6 and alpha lipoic acid. These vitamins can also help your diabetic neuropathy.

You need to prevent fat-soluble vitamin deficiency, especially vitamin D. Other lipid soluble vitamins are A, E and K. If possible, please take supplements for these. You might also develop thiamine and folate deficiency. Therefore, it is important to keep supplementing your diet with these vitamins.

My doctor put me on a medication called metoclopramide. When I read the side effects, they are very severe. Should I continue taking it?

This is the first-line of treatment for gastroparesis. It is a dopamine 2 receptor antagonist, a 5-HT 4 agonist, and a weak 5-HT3 receptor antagonist. It improves gastric emptying by enhancing gastric annular contractions and decreases postprandial gastric fundal relaxation. It is true that after long-term use this medication can have serious side effects. These side effects may include anxiety, restlessness, depression, hyperprolacti-nemia, QT interval prolongation and a condition called dyskinesia. Dyskinesia is characterized by involuntary movements of the tongue, lips, face, trunk and extremities.
You indeed must talk to your doctor if you need to take this medication on a long-term basis.

Domperidone was recommended to me, but it is not FDA approved in the US. Where can I buy it?

Domperidone is still not FDA approved since it can cause sudden death. It is recommended that you have an EKG before and during the treatment. You need to stop if your corrected QT interval is >470 ms if you are a man and if >450 ms if you are a woman.
Domperidone has many drug interactions. It is legal in Canada, and many of my patients buy it from a Canadian online pharmacy. You need to talk to your doctor before you use it.

How can macrolide antibiotics help relieve gastroparesis?

Macrolide antibiotics, like erythromycin or azithromycin induces high-amplitude gastric propulsive contractions that increase gastric emptying.

Can I take macrolide antibiotics long term?

No, you should not. You should not take these longer than four weeks at a time.

What are the risks of using macrolide antibiotics?

Long-term antibiotic use can induce antibiotic resistant strains. It might also cause gastrointestinal toxicity, hearing damage, or sudden death due to QT prolongation.

Why is cisapride not readily available in US?

Cisapride is a 5HT4 agonist which stimulates gastral and duodenal motility and accelerates gastric emptying of solids and liquids. Cisapride is better tolerated than metoclopramide, but its use has been associated with sudden death.

Why does my sugar vary widely from very low to very high?

Gastroparesis can make your diabetes control a nightmare, especially for someone with type 1 diabetes. Food that stays in the stomach is not digested, and their sugar might drop if their insulin is not adjusted properly.

Gastroparesis can also cause diabetic ketoacidosis that makes your nausea and vomiting worse. I have seen this happen in patients with type 1 diabetes when their sugar was not high and no insulin was given, or because they were not eating and no insulin was given, or not enough insulin was given. Because of nausea and vomiting, they are not drinking fluid and develop severe dehydration. The patient then develops diabetic ketoacidosis. The nausea and vomiting itself can also cause or worsen diabetic ketoacidosis.

Food that stays in the stomach too long might spoil and cause bacteria to grow and cause food poisoning. This can make the nausea and vomiting even worse.

Undigested food can harden and form a lump or a ball that is called a bezoar. This can cause obstructions which cause worsening nausea and vomiting.

Dehydration causes an electrolyte imbalance and may cause insulin resistance. Then, your sugar might go sky high.

What can we do about my unstable sugar?

If you have type 1 diabetes, you certainly are using insulin. Do not use any Amylin product. Any long-acting insulin is recommended. For fast-acting insulin, I recommend that you use regular insulin instead of analogs like Humalog, Novolog or Apidra. Regular insulin might match your prolonged food retention in the stomach.
Any time before you eat, check your sugar, and give a bolus properly.
If you have type 2 diabetes, stopping all oral medication is recommended. No oral medication is good for you. I recommended you start insulin also. Here are the reasons: metformin might cause worsening of your gastroparesis. SGLT2 antagonists cause dehydration which might lead to DKA. However, if you do not have vomiting and can tolerate fluids. SGLT2 antagonists can be tried. Sulphonylurea might cause severe hypoglycemia.

Check your sugar every time before you eat or when you feel your sugar is too high or too low.

Ideally, to stabilize your sugar you need an insulin pump and a CGM. We can use the special features of your pump to stabilize your sugar, and we can use CGM to monitor your sugar more closely.

Chapter 17: Diabetic foot care and diabetic neuropathy

Why should I check my feet every day?

Most diabetics have diabetic neuropathy and you can have a problem even before you realize it. At least 50% of amputations occur in diabetic patients and are due to infected diabetic foot ulcer. Before it is too late, you need to check your feet every day. It is an important part of diabetes self-care.

I cannot see the bottom of my feet. What can I do?

Before going to bed or after a shower ask your loved one to check for you, or you can use a mirror. This does not take too long.

What daily foot care should I do?

You need to wash your feet with mild soap and warm water. Soaking your feet is not recommended since it might increase your chance of infection. It is very important to test the water temperature. It should be warm, not hot. Then dry your feet thoroughly including between your toes.

Why are my feet very dry and cracked?

This is because you have diabetic neuropathy, which causes the sweat glands not to work properly.

What brand is the best cream or moisturizer for diabetic dry feet?

Most patients who use Eucerin or Gold Bond Ultimate are satisfied. I have patients who use O'Keeffe's foot cream and have positive reviews. Coconut oil is very good too and it is natural.

What should I do if I find a small cut or scratches on my foot?

Again, if it is small, and if there is no sign of infection like severe redness, swelling or oozing secretion or pus, then you can wash it with clean warm water and a very gentle soap. Do this for the whole foot and dry it well. Look carefully any debris in the cut. If you see some debris, use a tweezers sterilized with alcohol to remove it. Apply a very thin layer of antibiotic cream like Neosporin, Polysporin or Bactroban. Then cover it with a bandage.

What should I do if I have a deep cut?

If you have any deep cut or any small cut on your foot, and you do not feel like you should take care of it yourself, go see your doctor or podiatrist.

When should I get a tetanus shot?

If you have a deep cut and your last tetanus shot was 5 years ago, you should talk to your doctor and get one.

What is the most important thing to do to prevent future cuts?

Examine the cut and think about it. Try to figure out why you got the cut in the first place. You need to have a pair of good shoes and good socks. You might be qualified to get a pair of diabetic shoes which can be fitted for you. Talk to your doctor and see a podiatrist.

When should I see a doctor for a cut?

You should see a doctor whenever you feel you need to see a doctor. Please trust your gut and see one. You should see a doctor when you have a deep cut, especially with redness, swelling, pain or a wound oozing with pus. You should see a doctor for any wound you managed yourself and then it did not get better.

I have a blister on my foot. What should I do?

If the blister is small, look carefully at your shoes to see if anything there caused it, and do not wear that shoe again. You need to see a podiatrist to make sure your shoes and socks are a good fit for you. If the blister is small, you do not need to drain it. It will be absorbed in a few days as long as the cause is removed.
However, if the blister is big, and if there is a good chance it will break on its own, I recommend you drain the blister.
Here's how:

1. Wash your hands and the blister with soap and warm water. Swab the blister with iodine if you have it. It is okay if you do not have it. You can use 70% alcohol.
2. Find a clean, sharp unused needle.
3. Use the needle to puncture the blister. Aim for several spots near the blister's edge. Let the fluid drain, but leave the overlying skin in place.
4. Apply an ointment (Vaseline, Plastibase, Bactroban, Neosporin, or others) to the blister and cover it with a nonstick gauze bandage. If a rash appears, stop using the ointment.
5. Change the dressing every day. Apply more ointment and a bandage.

I have calluses. What should I do?

A callus is not something you should take care of yourself, since if not properly taken care of, it might lead to infection and a foot ulcer. Go to see a podiatrist and let a professional take care of it. The podiatrist will help you to get a pair of therapeutic diabetic shoes and good support inserts. These will prevent future calluses.

I just found an ulcer on my foot. What should I do?

If you had followed my instructions for foot care, you might not have one today. Hopefully, this is your wake-up call to check your sugar and eat right to get your sugar in better control.
First, you need to keep it clean and see a podiatrist for wound care as soon as you can. Based on the severity, you might need antibiotics, wound cleaning, debridement, and off-loading. There is no way you can take care of an ulcer yourself. You need to see a doctor. This is really important if you have fever or oozing pus. The ulcer might cause a blood infection or a bone infection, and it needs to be taken care of by a doctor as soon as you can.

No matter what I do, I have freezing cold feet. Is there anything you can suggest?

Cold feet can be very annoying and cold feet can decrease your quality of life. Your feet can feel cold even when the rest of your body is very hot. I call it "cold feet syndrome." A small fraction of patients has vascular problems (circulation problems), but most people have diabetic neuropathy.

First, you can try Capsaicin cream. You can buy it from drugstores like CVS or Walgreens. If this is not effective, your doctor might try Gabapentin or Lyrica. Wearing warm socks always helps, but usually this cannot solve the problem.

Here is one thing you should never do. Do not stick your feet in hot water that might burn your feet and cause infection. It is okay to warm your feet with warm water bottles and heating pads with appropriate temperature.

If you have a circulation problem with the big vessels in your feet, we call this peripheral vascular disease. We can test for this and confirm it. If you have small vessel disease we cannot even test for it.

If the above measures are not effective, your doctor should test you for peripheral vascular disease and treat it accordingly, especially if you have pain and it becomes worse after walking.

I have found that I have a black toe. What should I do?

Hopefully, you knew this before. Diabetic vascular problems, such as peripheral vascular disease, can cause an ulcer or gangrene. Sometimes when this happens, amputation is the only solution. Therefore, take care of yourself. Check your sugar and take your medications as prescribed. Do not wait until it is too late.

Can you reiterate when I should see my doctor immediately?

You should see your doctor if any of the following situation occurs:
- You developed an open wound, or ulceration with or without infection.
- New developed neuropathy pain or pain at rest.
- Mid foot pain especially with red, hot or swollen.
- Diminished pulse on your foot.
- Your foot becomes purple or blue.
- You have a black toe.

I have diabetic neuropathy and I have burning pain in my feet. It is so bad that I cannot sleep. What should I do?

Diabetic neuropathy can be very challenging to treat and can significantly reduce your quality of life. Therefore, I always recommend to my patients that they should care for their diabetes seriously.

Here are some things you can do to help your neuropathy:
1. Your doctor should do a careful foot exam to make sure there are no other foot complications. Make sure there are no other conditions besides diabetes that would worsen your diabetic neuropathy. Many diabetes patients also have heart failure, obesity and vein insufficiency. These can cause severe bilateral low extremity swelling. The swelling can compromise the small vessel circulation and worsen the neuropathy. The swelling needs to be treated. Otherwise, the other measures might not be effective.
2. I would try some over the counter vitamins, such as B12, B6 and lipoic acid.
3. If this is still not working, I would try a prescription vitamin like Metanx which contains an active form of folic acid and vitamins B6 and B12.
4. If this is still not effective, I would try Gabapentin or Lyrica.
5. Some patients have found SSRI or SNRI to be helpful.
6. I have patients who have used all of above but still cannot get relief.
7. Lidocaine spray can be tried. Other creams like Capsaicin might also be used as an adjunctive treatment.

I have chronic diabetic wound. I have been seeing a wound doctor, but it is not healing. What can I do?

Sometimes, It can be very difficult to heal for a few reasons. Your sugar might not be under control. You might not have good circulation. You might have secondary infection which is hard to control. Sometimes amputation has to be done.

Is there any supplement do you recommend promoting wound healing?

Lots supplements are claimed to be helpful, but there are no good studies to prove it. However, I think it might be helpful to take some vitamin A (small amount), vitamin C, vitamin D, iron, copper, zinc, and some essential amino acids like arginine, glutamine and leucine, etc.

Again, taking care of your diabetes is the best way to avoid all these troubles.

Chapter 18: Diabetes and sexual dysfunction

How common is the problem of sexual dysfunction in men with diabetes?

The likelihood of having difficulty with an erection occurs in approximately 50% to 60% of men with diabetes for men over 50. Above age 70, there is about a 95% likelihood of having some difficulty with erectile dysfunction.

Why do men with diabetes have erectile dysfunction?

Successful erections need the nerves and blood vessels to work together. If the nerves or blood vessels have problems, it will lead to erectile dysfunction. As we know, long-term diabetes can cause diabetic neuropathy and cardiovascular disease.

I am over 60, why should I care about sex?

It is normal to have slightly reduced libido as you age, but even men in their 90s can still have normal sexual function. Sexual dysfunction can affect your mood, motivation, self-esteem and relationships profoundly. As we discussed above, erectile dysfunction can be a sign of cardiovascular disease. You might also need to alert your doctor and be tested for this.

I am embarrassed. How should I raise this issue with my doctor?

Your doctor should ask this question, but more often, he or she does not. Your doctor is being pressed by Medicare and the insurance companies to treat more patients. The insurance companies are less concerned about patient wellbeing than your doctor. Your doctor's time is focused on your blood pressure, cholesterol, blood sugar, and A1c.

You need to be your own advocate and raise this issue to your doctor if he or she does not ask you about it.

As we discussed above, you are not alone. If you are above 50 and have had diabetes for at least 10 years, your chance of having ED is over 50%. So, just be direct with your doctor and tell him or her that you have ED.

What can I do to prevent ED?

Here are a few things you can do:
1. Try your best to work with your doctor to get your diabetes under control. There is a direct correlation between the A1c and ED.
2. Stop smoking if you are a smoker.
3. Make diet, exercise and life-style changes to make sure your weight is under control.
4. Take your statins as prescribed.

Should I stop drinking?

Yes, you should. Alcohol can cause ED or make ED worse.

What should I do if I have ED?

Here are seven recommendations:
1. Raise this issue with your doctor, as we discussed. This might indicate you have a more serious condition like cardiovascular disease. Your doctor might refer you to a cardiologist to have a test.
2. Stop smoking. If you smoke, it's never too late to quit.
3. Talk to your partner. Help your partner understand this can be caused by diabetes or cardiovascular disease. Let your partner know you are struggling with it. Tell your partner this is not because you have less love, or that your sexual needs are being met from somewhere else. Your partner's understanding and support plays a very important part in making sure you can succeed.
4. Ask your doctor to review your medications. There is a long list of medications that can cause or worsen ED. Some medications may be able to be discontinued or changed.
5. Get the gear to get yourself in shape.
6. Try your best to follow a good diabetic regimen to get it under control.

7. You might ask to try medications like sildenafil (generic Viagra), Viagra, Levitra, Cialis, Stendra, etc.

Is there anything else I can do if my insurance does not pay for Viagra, Levitra, Stendra, or Cialis?

It is sad now how your insurance dictates your treatment. The good news is Viagra is now generic. It is available as sildenafil (20 mg per tab). You can ask your doctor for it. It is not available in all pharmacies.

How do I use sildenafil?

Sildenafil is 20 mg per tab. I recommend taking 1 tab ½-4 hr before sexual activity. If not effective, next time, you can increase the dose to 2 tabs, up to 4 tabs.

Can I buy ED drugs online?

The standard answer is NO. Apparently you are running a risk of not getting the pure medication, not the right dose, contamination and all sorts of other issues. You may not know what you are truly taking. Again, nowadays, due to the insurance, patients are being squeezed and pushed. I understand your pain. You have to take your own risks. I have anecdotal evidence for both sides of the issue.

Are there any herbs I can try?

There is no standard trial to confirm any herbs work for this purpose. The common supplements people are trying are:
1. Ginkgo biloba is an herb from a Chinese tree. Your risk for bleeding may increase, especially if you are on blood thinning medications. So do not start this on your own. You need to talk to your doctor before you start.
2. Ginseng is very popular in Asia, especially, in China.
3. Rhodiola Rosea.
4. L-arginine is an amino acid which is the substrate to make nitric oxide. This is the gas which was found to relax penis blood vessels. The effectiveness and side effects have not been well-defined.

Acupuncture is known to stimulate the nerves which are important to regulate penis blood supply.

What do I need to know before I try prescription medications like sildenafil, Viagra, Levitra, Stendra, and Cialis?

If you have cardiovascular disease and you are taking nitrates, you should not take them. It might cause very severe low blood pressure which could be life threatening. The same thing is true if you have taken an ED medication in the past 24 hours. If you have chest pain, make sure you tell the physician who is treating you.
Other side effects include, but are not limited to, headaches, flushing, nasal congestion, indigestion and vision impairment.

Should I have my doctor check my testosterone?

Testosterone certainly plays a very important role in sexual function. It is extremely important for libido. It also has a permissive role for erection.
The decrease in testosterone in diabetes is mostly due to secondary causes. You may have depression, chronic pain, obstructive sleep apnea, stress, or poor sleep. The medications used to treat these and other conditions might reduce your testosterone. Also, testosterone is converted to estrogen in fat cells by an enzyme called aromatase.
It is very reasonable to have your doctor check your testosterone.

When should I check my testosterone?

You should have your doctor check your testosterone early in the morning. Testosterone secretion has a diurnal pattern. It is highest early in the morning.

My testosterone was at a low level. Should I get it treated?

You should be evaluated by an endocrinologist. Please do not go to a testosterone clinic. I personally found at least five pituitary tumors which were being wrongly treated with injectable testosterone. This is beyond the discussion of this book.

Chapter 19: More questions about diabetes emergencies

How to prevent low sugar and how to treat low sugar have been discussed in other chapters in this book. Here we are going to focus on two other diabetic emergencies—diabetes ketoacidosis (DKA) and hyperosmolar hyperglycemic state (HHS).

What is diabetic ketoacidosis?

Our body needs a certain acid level, hydration and electrolytes to work properly. Our body is amazing. It can keep all of these in a balanced status under normal conditions.

Normally, our body breaks down sugar as a source of energy. In this process, insulin is required. As you now know in type 1 diabetes, insulin is deficient. If our body does not have enough insulin, then our body cannot use sugar and our body will break down fat for our energy. The problem is that it breaks down too much and exceeds our body's ability to use them. The product of fat breakdown is ketones which is acid. Too much ketone buildup in the body is toxic. They make your body very acidic which makes your body not work properly. They (the ketones) and increased sugar also drag out lots water from your body which make your body very dehydrated. Diabetic ketoacidosis is a serious problem. It can happen to people with either type 1 or type 2 diabetes, but it is more likely to affect people with type 1.

What is the mortality rate for DKA?

DKA is a serious complication of diabetes associated with significant mortality and high healthcare costs. The overall DKA mortality in the US is less than 1%, but a rate higher than 5% is reported in the elderly and in patients with concomitant, life-threatening illnesses.

What other damage might DKA do to your body?

DKA is an emergency. Many long-term effects have not been well-studied, but evidence has shown that repeated DKAs certainly damage a patient's brain and also increase long-term MACE (major adverse cardiac events).

Mortality in patients with HHS is reported between 5% and 16%, which is about 10 times higher than the mortality in patients with DKA.

What causes diabetic ketoacidosis?

People can get diabetic ketoacidosis for a few reasons:

1. **It is not known that you have diabetes.** Quite a high percentage of patients are diagnosed with type 1diabetes because they are presented as DKA. A study from Colorado data between 1998 and 2012 determined diabetic ketoacidosis was present in 1,339 of 3,439 youth (38.9%) at type 1 diabetes diagnosis. Youth with DKA had a median age of 9.4 years (interquartile range, 5.6-12.6 years), 53.8% were male, and 75.7% were white.

2. **Patients forget to take insulin**. I also have patients who cannot pay for insulin, or they just do not take it when they should.

3. **Patients do not check their sugar**. If sugar is not checked regularly, and patients do not give insulin or do not give enough insulin.

4. **Insulin pump failure.** This also includes user errors such as not changing an infusion set or kinked tubing, or scar formation at the insertion site and gastrointestinal infection.

5. **Major health problem.** The patient might have a major illness or health problem, such as a heart attack or infection.

6. **Taking certain medicines or illegal drugs.**

7. **Patients do not take their insulin as directed.**

8. **Taking an SGLT2 medication.** Now, we have a new type 2 diabetes medication called SGLT2 inhibitors (see other section for details); The FDA warns that this category of medication might cause type 2 diabetes to have normal sugar DKA.

110

What are the symptoms of diabetic ketoacidosis?

The symptoms can include but are not limited to the following, and the patient can have some or all of them. Symptoms can also start gradually and get worse Including:
1. Feeling very thirsty and drinking a lot of water.
2. Urinating a lot, including at night.
3. Nausea or vomiting is very common.
4. Belly pain.
5. Feeling tired or having trouble thinking clearly.
6. Having breath that smells sweet or fruity.
7. If severe enough and not treated, patients can have confusion and loss of consciousness and even death.

Should I see a doctor?

This is a life-threatening emergency. You need to go to the ER.

Is there anything I can do to prevent diabetic ketoacidosis?

Yes. Here are six recommendations for preventing DKA.
1. Take care of your diabetes. Eat and exercise right and take your insulin as prescribed.
2. Monitor your blood sugar levels. This is the key to keeping you out of trouble. You also need to have a plan to react to your high and low readings. If you do not have a plan, talk to your doctor.
3. Adjust your insulin dosage as needed. Again, it is very good for you to check your sugar, but is just as important that you need to know what to do about these numbers. Please see my other sections, about how to respond to high sugar.
4. Check your ketone level. When you are ill or under stress, test your urine for excess ketones with an over-the-counter urine ketone test kit. If your ketone level is moderate or high, especially if you have other symptoms of DKA (see above), you definitely need to go to the ER.
5. If you have type 2 diabetes, and if you are taking one of the new SGLT2 inhibitor medications, you need to stop your medication and keep yourself well-hydrated. When you go to the ER, you need to let your treating physician know what you are taking.
6. Know what medication you have to take and what medication you can stop temporarily. When your doctor starts you on a new

medication, you need to know when you need to stop and when you should not stop taking it.

How is diabetic ketoacidosis treated?

You need to go to the hospital to be treated.

- **Replenish fluids and correct electrolytes**. In DKA, patients lose a lot of fluid and also have electrolyte disturbances.
- **Take Insulin.** When the body has enough insulin, your body will start to use sugar as fuel and suppress your body from producing more ketones. Gradually your excess ketones will be metabolized and the acidic condition will be corrected.

What is a hyperosmolar hyperglycemic state (HHS)?

A hyperosmolar hyperglycemic state is another life-threatening diabetic emergency. This mostly occurs in type 2 diabetes patients. Our bodies are designed to have everything balanced and maintained in a very narrow normal range.

If the sugar gets too high, the sugar will pull water out of the cells and out of the body. This can cause the body's metabolism to be severely deranged.

What are the symptoms of a hyperosmolar hyperglycemic state?

A hyperosmolar hyperglycemic state can cause severe fatigue, disorientation, passing out (losing consciousness) and coma. But before that happens, people usually have symptoms for a few days that include:

- Urinating much more than usual
- Being very thirsty, and drinking much more than usual
- Losing weight
- Having dark yellow or brown urine

What are the factors which can cause a hyperosmolar hyperglycemic state?

HHS can be caused by several factors:

112

- Getting an infection or severe fever illness, especially a GI tract illness. This will usually cause nausea, vomiting and diarrhea.

- Having a heart attack or stroke.

- Stopping diabetes medicines or not taking the diabetes medicines as directed.

- Taking other medicines that affect sugar levels like high dose steroids.

- Becoming dehydrated. This is when the body loses too much water.

Is there a test for a hyperosmolar hyperglycemic state?

Yes.

Regularly check your sugar. If your sugar is consistently higher than 500, and you are not able to get it down, you need to go to hospital. The hospital will do the tests to determine if you are in a hyperosmolar hyperglycemic state.

What can I do to prevent a hyperosmolar hyperglycemic state?

1. Take care of your diabetes. Eat and exercise right and take your insulin or your oral medications as prescribed.

2. Monitor your blood sugar levels. This is the key to keeping you out of trouble. You also need to have a plan to react to your readings. If you do not have a plan, talk to your doctor. It is also very important to know under what circumstances you need to stop taking certain medications.

3. Adjust your insulin dosage as needed. If you are taking insulin, it is important to know what you can do to get your sugar down under certain circumstances. Again, it is very good for you to check your sugar, but it is as important that you know what you should do about these numbers. Please see my other section, about how to respond to high sugar.

4. Check your ketone levels. A hyperosmolar hyperglycemic state usually occurs in adults with type 2 diabetes, but you need to check your ketones, too. When you are ill or under stress, test your urine for excess ketones with an over-the-counter urine ketones test kit. If your ketone level is

113

moderate or high, especially if you have other symptoms of HHS (see above), you definitely need to go to the ER.

5. When you have high sugar and shortness of breath, chest pain and you feel very sick, you certainly need to go to the ER

6. Know what medication you have to take and what medication you can stop temporarily. When your doctor starts you on a new medication, you need to know when you need to stop taking it, and when you should not stop taking it.

7. Always keep yourself well hydrated.

8. If you have a GI tract disease or gastroparesis, and if you are not able to keep water and food down, you need to go to see your doctor as soon as possible. You are usually given IV fluids which can prevent you from getting into full-blown hyperosmolar hyperglycemic state.

How is a hyperosmolar hyperglycemic state treated?

Patients with a hyperosmolar hyperglycemic state are treated in the hospital. These patients have severe dehydration and electrolyte disturbances.

- Fluids and electrolytes – In a hyperosmolar hyperglycemic state, the body loses a lot of fluids.

- Insulin is also given intravenously to get the sugar down slowly.

- The doctor will also treat any infection or illness causing the hyperosmolar hyperglycemic state.

Final Words

What are your final words on diabetes?

You actually have a big part to play in taking care of your diabetes. It is not all up to your doctor. You have the biggest part to play in taking care of your diabetes. This can be very challenging. However, there are many things you can do to make diabetes self-care work for you.

The ADA (American Diabetes Association) recommends the following seven self-care guidelines. If you follow these guidelines, you will greatly improve your overall diabetes care results.

1. **Healthy eating.** This is absolutely the most important of the seven. If your eating is not fixed, your diabetes can never be controlled no matter what medications you use. As I discussed, I recommend a low-meat, low-carb, high-fiber diet.

2. **Being active**. Being active is not just exercising. What I mean is that if you can stand, do not sit. If you can move around, do not stand still. Keep moving and do activities that require moving like cleaning, gardening, cooking, shopping, etc.

3. **Monitoring.** Check your sugar as recommended. Check your ketones as needed. Check your blood pressure as required. Also, make sure your doctor monitors your A1c, cholesterol, urine protein, etc.

4. **Taking medications**. Take the medications you are supposed to take, and know when and why you need to take them. If you are not taking the medications you are supposed to take, this can mislead your treating doctor. This might cause your doctor to make the wrong assumptions and hurt you eventually. I have a patient who is supposed to take long-acting insulin every day, but he did not follow the regimen due to financial difficulties. He took his insulin every other day. His sugar was not controlled, and then his doctor increased his insulin all the way to over 300 units daily. His sugar was up and down. If, for some reason, you cannot take

your medication as you are supposed to, you need to let your treating doctor know, and the regimen or medication needs to be changed. Your doctor can help you make the right changes.

5. **Risk reduction.** If you are a smoker, strive to quit. Make sure you have a yearly dilated eye exam. Check your own feet every day. Have regular podiatrist visits. Have all the vaccines you are supposed to have, like a yearly flu vaccine. Other vaccines like hepatitis B, pneumonia and shingles are also recommended for patients at different ages.

6. **Problem solving.** Life is complicated. Life is even more complicated with diabetes. Strive to learn problem-solving skills. Different problems pop up all the time. Try to learn about diabetes as much as possible, so you can manage it better. Then you will not have to be panic when difficult situations arise.

7. **Healthy coping.** Again, dealing with diabetes is very challenging, and it is normal to have different emotions. Make sure you do not to let depression, frustration or anxiety affect you management of diabetes.

Subscribe to our YouTube channel

DrBaoEndoClinic

www.ingramcontent.com/pod-product-compliance
Lightning Source LLC
Chambersburg PA
CBHW020209200326
41521CB00005BA/305